TACTICAL INTIMACY

THE TIS METHOD. THE SCIENCE OF LASTING LONGER, CONFIDENT PERFORMANCE, AND DEEP INTIMATE CONNECTION FOR MEN

ERDEM ERGIN

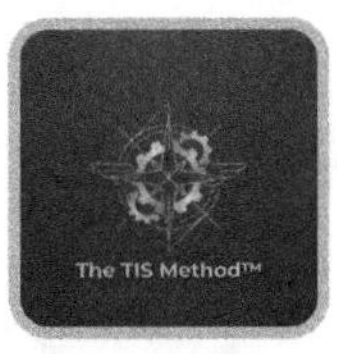

TIS METHOD

First Edition: 2026

Published by TIS Method

Paperback ISBN: 979-8-9953572-0-9

Hardcover ISBN: 979-8-9953572-1-6

eBook ISBN: 979-8-9953572-2-3

Visit our official website: www.tismethod.com

For permissions, bulk orders, or media inquiries: info@tismethod.com

Available in print and digital editions

*To every man who has ever felt the gap
between who he is and who he knows he could be.*

And to the partners who stand beside them.

Contents

Introduction: The Operator's Manual You Should Have Been Given

Is it too late to upgrade the most important system in your life?

NOT YOUR CAREER. NOT your finances. Not your fitness routine. The system that governs how you show up in your most intimate moments. The system that determines whether your partner feels cherished or tolerated, connected or merely serviced. The system that, whether you realize it or not, echoes through every domain of your existence.

A truth most men never discover: the control you achieve in the bedroom does not stay in the bedroom. The man who masters his body's most primal responses becomes the man who masters his schedule, his finances, his health, his relationships. And the reverse is equally true: the chaos you tolerate in your intimate life will bleed into everything else. Anxiety breeds anxiety. Frustration compounds. The feeling of being out of control in one arena quietly infects every other.

This book will teach you to interrupt that cycle.

Within these pages, you will find a complete system for achieving what most men have given up hoping for: reliable, repeatable control over your body's timing. Not through numbing creams that steal sensation. Not through distraction techniques that disconnect you from your partner. Through a mechanical, trainable protocol that works with your biology, not against it.

But lasting longer is only the beginning. The same principles that give you command in the bedroom, breath regulation, nervous system mastery, strategic patience, will transform how you move through the world. You will become more present with your partner, more patient with your children, more focused in your work, more intentional with your time. The man who chooses when to finish becomes the man who chooses how to live.

Your partner will notice the difference. Not just in duration, but in presence. In attention. In the quality of connection that most couples lose after the first year and never recover. You will become, in the truest sense, irreplaceable.

This is not a book of cheap tricks. This is the *Operator's Manual* for the most important system you own. A system built on engineering principles, not a grab bag of flimsy tips. Written for the man who has achieved real success in other domains of his life, in his career, his fitness, or his finances, through discipline, strategy, and an unrelenting desire to understand how things actually work.

And yet, in the most intimate and arguably most important arena of his life, this same man often feels like a complete novice.

This is the great unspoken paradox of the modern successful man. The very mental and neurological wiring that makes you formidable in business can turn you into a rookie in the bedroom. The mindset that allows you to dominate your professional world, with its speed, laser focus, and ruthless efficiency, is precisely what sabotages you in the one arena that demands a different kind of control. A different form of patience. A deep capacity for connection.

Whether you are a CEO navigating high-stakes negotiations, a young professional climbing the ladder, an entrepreneur building something from nothing, or simply a man who refuses to accept "average" in any area that matters, this paradox likely resonates. This book is the roadmap to resolving it.

We will deconstruct the single most common and least discussed male sexual challenge: premature ejaculation and the performance anxiety that feeds it. But let me be clear from the start. We are not here to "fix a problem." We are here to master a skill.

The reframe matters. This is not a personal failure to be ashamed of. It is a technical issue with a clear, engineering-based solution.

The *Tactical Intimacy System* (*TIS*) is a teachable, evidence-informed philosophy that synthesizes physiological control, mental focus, and emotional connection.

It is purpose-built for the modern, analytical mind. We do not traffic in vague concepts. We deal in actionable, science-based protocols that work directly on your neurology and physiology.

Think of it this way: we will open the hood of your own machine, identify the control mechanisms that have been running on autopilot for years, and teach you how to operate them with the same deliberate mastery you bring to your professional life.

Throughout these pages, you will move through a three-stage transformation:

1. From *Predator* to *Commander*. You will learn to shift your mental objective from a frantic, goal-fixated sprint to a calm, pleasure-centered mission, eliminating performance anxiety at its root.

2. From *Commander* to *Pilot*. You will master the *TIS Engine*: the synthesis of breath, muscle, and rhythm that puts you in conscious control of your body's responses.

3. From *Pilot* to *Artist*. You will learn to wield your newfound control not merely to last longer, but to become a virtuoso of mutual pleasure, capable of creating and sustaining extraordinary intimate connection with your partner.

This journey demands discipline. It requires practice. The man who internalizes the principles in this book will not only transform his intimate life. He will find that the same skills transfer outward. He will become calmer under pressure, more present in conversations, more confident in situations that once triggered anxiety.

You have already demonstrated you can achieve mastery in one world. Now it is time to bring that same capacity to the arena that matters most.

A Note on the Men in This Book

When I first developed the techniques in this book, I did not keep them to myself.

Over the course of several months, I shared what I had learned with three men I trusted: my neighbor, a fellow parent I had met through our sons' school, and a close friend whose marriage had hit a rough patch. Each was struggling with the same challenge I had faced. Each was skeptical that anything could help. And each agreed to try the system, on one condition: I would document their progress.

What happened next became the foundation of this book.

Their names have been changed to protect their privacy, but their stories are real. Their struggles are real. And their transformations are documented throughout these pages, not as hypothetical examples, but as proof that this system works for men at different ages, in different life stages, facing different challenges.

John is 28, a software engineer, in a relationship with his girlfriend. He is the younger man navigating career pressure and modern dating.

Matt is 38, a trauma surgeon, married with a young son and daughter. He is the high-achieving professional whose demanding work leaves little room for presence at home.

David is 41, a construction project manager, married for 15 years with a teenage daughter. He is the established man seeking to reignite a long-term relationship and build a lasting legacy.

You will follow their journeys through every chapter. You will see them struggle, adapt, and ultimately transform. You will witness their conversations with their partners, their physical transformations, their breakthroughs and setbacks.

By the end, you will understand that their success is not exceptional. It is replicable. What worked for John, Matt, and David will work for you.

Welcome to *Tactical Intimacy: The TIS Method*.

CHAPTER 1

THE APEX PREDATOR PARADOX

The View from the Top

THE GLASS WALL OF the conference room overlooks a city that sprawls beneath you, a kingdom of concrete and light, humming with a million separate lives you will never know. Inside, the air is thick with tension, a currency you trade as comfortably as stocks. You have been in this negotiation for three hours. Your opponents are tired; you can see it in the way they shift in their chairs, in the subtle slump of their shoulders. Their arguments are frayed. You are not. You are energized by this environment. Your mind is a laser, cutting through the noise, anticipating their next move before they have even formulated it. With a final, calm, and calculated statement, you do not just win; you dominate. The deal is closed. As you shake hands, feeling the limp, defeated grip of your adversary, your pulse is steady, your mind already processing the next three steps to execute the plan. In the concrete jungle of the modern world, you are the apex predator. This is your superpower.

Hours later, you are in a different room. The lights are low, the ambiance is intimate. The person across from you is not an opponent to be conquered, but a partner to connect with. And yet, the steady calm you commanded just hours ago has vanished. A different kind of tension fills the air, and this time, it is not your ally. The laser-like focus is replaced by a frantic internal monologue of doubt. *Am I doing this right? Is she enjoying this? Do not finish too soon. Do not mess this up.* The predator has become the prey to his own anxiety. The man who can command a boardroom is now lost in his own head, a spectator at his own life's most intimate event.

Where does that superpower go when you close the bedroom door?

This is the disconnect that no one talks about: the very same mental and neural wiring that makes you a titan in business can turn you into a novice in intimacy. This is the *Apex Predator Paradox*.

The Silent Statistic That Binds Us

Consider a number that most men feel but rarely discuss. According to research published in the *Journal of Sexual Medicine*, approximately one in three men report experiencing premature ejaculation at some point in their lives.

One in three.

Look around your next board meeting, your gym, your group of high-achieving friends. The odds are that this silent frustration is a shared reality, a deeply personal struggle fought in isolation. Consider the men in that conference room with you. Statistically, at least one of them is fighting the same battle, projecting an image of unflappable control while privately wrestling with a profound sense of failure. This erodes confidence, creates distance in relationships, and turns what should be a source of connection into a source of dread.

Most men miss a critical point: for high-achieving men, the leaders and deal-makers who thrive on pressure and control, that number is often perceived to be even higher. Why? Because their entire identity is built on performance and successful outcomes. A missed sales target and a premature orgasm can trigger the same deep-seated fear of failure. This is not a failure of biology. It is a catastrophic failure of programming. Your life has been an endless series of finish lines to cross, and your nervous system has become ruthlessly efficient at getting there.

This book will teach you to override that programming. It will not ask you to change who you are or to abandon the drive that made you successful. It will teach you how to take the formidable power you already possess and wield it in the one arena where it seems to fail you.

You are about to understand why that "predator" instinct, the very thing that got you to the top, works against you in an arena that demands a different kind of control, a different form of patience, and a deep sense of connection. You will see that the problem is not you; the problem is your operating system trying to execute the wrong program in the wrong environment.

Your Two Operating Systems: The Hunter and the Lover

The paradox has a root cause: your nervous system runs on two fundamental, and often competing, operating systems. For millions of years, these systems were balanced by the natural rhythms of life. In the modern world, with its constant notifications, deadlines, and pressures, for men like you, that balance has been destroyed.

The Hunter's OS (The Sympathetic Nervous System)

This is your *Fight or Flight* mode. Think of it as the high-performance operating system that kicks in when you are hunting a target. Whether that target is a quarterly sales goal, a hostile takeover, or a literal wildebeest on the savanna, the biological response is the same. Your brain identifies a target and an objective: *close that deal, win that argument, solve that problem.* Instantly, it floods your system with cortisol, adrenaline, and norepinephrine.

It is a Formula 1 car: built for speed, aggression, and the finish line. It burns high-octane fuel and is designed for one purpose: to win the race as quickly as possible.

Your heart rate increases, sending more oxygen to your muscles. Your pupils dilate, sharpening your focus on the target. Your blood flow is redirected from non-essential functions, such as digestion, immune response, or nuanced emotional processing, to your limbs. Your mind becomes a ruthlessly efficient, linear processor. Fast, aggressive, and results-oriented.

Modern corporate and competitive life has conditioned you to live almost exclusively in this mode. Your phone buzzes with an urgent email, and you get a hit of adrenaline. You see a problem in a spreadsheet, and your mind immediately jumps to a solution. You are a finely tuned, target-acquiring machine. You are perpetually "on," running hot, ready for the next challenge.

This mode, when it is your only mode, is poison for intimacy. It is an operating system designed for conflict, not connection.

The Lover's OS (The Parasympathetic Nervous System)

This is your *Rest and Digest* mode. If the Hunter's OS is a Formula 1 car, the Lover's OS is a luxury all-terrain vehicle, capable of navigating complex, beautiful landscapes with grace and patience. It enables trust, relaxation, sensory awareness, and the ability to lose yourself in the present moment. Its purpose is not to race to a destination, but to fully experience the journey.

This is the state required for deep connection, for savoring a fine meal, for listening intently to music, or for experiencing intimacy without a finish line. It is the system that allows you to feel the warmth of your partner's skin, to notice the subtle changes in her breathing, to be fully present in the shared space between you.

A predator on the hunt cannot be in Rest and Digest mode. He is always scanning the horizon, always anticipating the next move. And that is why the master of control in the boardroom can so easily lose control in the bedroom.

When you enter an intimate situation with the Hunter's OS still running, your body interprets it as another target-oriented mission. Your partner becomes the "target," orgasm becomes the "objective," and your nervous system does what it is trained to do: execute the mission as quickly and efficiently as possible.

The results? Premature ejaculation, performance anxiety, or that strange emotional disconnect you feel even in a moment of peak physical intensity. These are not your personal failures. They are the inevitable, predictable outcomes of trying to drive a high-performance race car on a winding, delicate country road. You keep crashing because you are using the wrong vehicle for the terrain, and the crash leaves behind damage for both you and your partner.

YOUR TWO OPERATING SYSTEMS

The Apex Predator Paradox: Why Your Greatest Strength Becomes Your Greatest Weakness

THE HUNTER'S OS	→ EVOLVE	THE LOVER'S OS
Sympathetic Nervous System		Parasympathetic Nervous System
Fast, goal-oriented — Sprint to the finish line		**Slow, process-oriented** — Savor the journey
Performance-driven — "How long did I last?"		**Pleasure-driven** — "How connected are we?"
Self-focused — Monitoring your own body		**Partner-focused** — Conducting her experience
Shallow breathing — Rapid, anxious, chest-level		**Coherence breathing** — Slow 5-5 count, diaphragmatic
Cortisol and adrenaline — Fight-or-flight hormones		**Oxytocin and dopamine** — Connection and reward hormones
Muscle tension — Pelvic floor clenching reflexively		**Controlled relaxation** — Pelvic floor fatigued by design
Result: Loss of control — Ejaculation within minutes		**Result: Complete command** — You choose when to finish

The TIS Method teaches you to switch operating systems at will.
The goal is not to kill the Hunter. It is to evolve him into a Commander.

Your Two Operating Systems

The Path Forward: From Predator to Pilot

The goal of this book, and the *Tactical Intimacy System,* is not to kill the predator within you. That predator is what makes you successful. It is a vital and powerful part of who you are. The goal is to give him a new set of tools, a new understanding of the terrain.

The goal is to evolve him.

Imagine a sniper. A novice thinks power is in the size of the bullet and the speed of firing. The master knows true power is in the absolute control of his own breath, the stillness of his body, and the precision of his execution. He can slow his heart rate on command, remain perfectly still under immense pressure, and execute with flawless precision at the exact moment he chooses. He is not a brute; he is a virtuoso of control. His power comes from restraint, not aggression.

We will take your power of focus and discipline and transform it from the brute force of a sprinter into the precision of a sniper. Instead of telling you "what to do" with a list of distractions, we will teach you how your system *actually* works. We will open the hood of your own machine, identify the control switches that have been dormant for years, and teach you how to operate them with the same mastery you apply to your business.

The man who commands a boardroom already has what it takes. He simply needs to learn a different kind of command.

Commander's Q&A: Your Initial Briefing

Is this just another book about performance anxiety?

No. Performance anxiety is a symptom, not the disease. The disease is a dysregulated nervous system stuck in Hunter mode. Most books try to treat the symptom with mental tricks that pull you further out of the moment. That is like trying to fix an overheating engine by turning up the radio to drown out the warning bells. We are going to fix the underlying mechanical problem. Once you learn how to control your physiological state, to consciously switch from the Hunter to the Lover OS, performance anxiety becomes irrelevant because its root cause has been eliminated.

I am successful because I am results-oriented. Are you telling me to stop being that way?

Absolutely not. We are going to channel that results-oriented mindset into a new, more sophisticated result. In business, you track Key Performance Indicators. Your old sexual KPI was likely "time to completion." We are going to upgrade your KPI to "Total Shared Experience." The objective is not changing; the definition of a successful outcome is getting a massive upgrade from a simple, binary goal to a rich, multi-faceted one that you are in complete control of.

How is this different from Tantra or other esoteric practices?

While we respect the wisdom of ancient traditions, as you will see in Chapter 3, the Tactical Intimacy System is built for the modern, analytical mind. We do not deal in vague concepts like "channeling energy." We deal in actionable, science-based protocols that work on your neurology and physiology. Tantra might ask you to *feel* the energy flow; we will show you the exact nerve pathways and hormonal responses that create that feeling and give you the controls to manage them. This is a system of engineering, not spirituality. It is for the man who wants to see the blueprint before he builds the house.

Is this not just overthinking something that should be natural and spontaneous?

Think of a world-class jazz musician. His improvisation seems completely natural and spontaneous, a magical flow of creativity. That spontaneity is only possible because he spent tens of thousands of hours practicing scales, learning music theory, and mastering his instrument until it became an extension of his body. The "natural" state you are experiencing now is likely dictated by anxiety and ingrained bad habits. It is an improvisation based on a limited skillset. By consciously mastering the fundamentals of your own "instrument," you create the foundation for true, confident, and exhilarating spontaneity to emerge.

What if I am not a "CEO" or "Apex Predator"? What if I am just a regular guy who wants more control?

The Apex Predator is a metaphor for a mindset that modern life forces upon all of us. Whether you are a lawyer, a software developer, a student, or an artist, you have been trained to be fast, efficient, and goal-oriented to survive and thrive. Our culture rewards the Hunter's OS. The paradox affects any man who feels a disconnect between his competence in the world and his control in the bedroom. This system is for any man who is ready to upgrade his programming.

Commander's Briefing: Chapter 1

- **The Apex Predator Paradox:** The same relentless, goal-oriented drive that makes you a titan in your career is the very programming that sabotages you in intimacy. Your greatest strength in one arena has become your greatest weakness in another.

- **You Have Two Operating Systems:** Your body is either in Hunter Mode (Sympathetic Nervous System), which is fast, aggressive, and built for a finish line, or Lover Mode (Parasympathetic Nervous System), which is calm, present, and built for connection. You have been stuck in Hunter Mode.

- **The Problem is Your Programming, Not You:** Your struggles with control and performance are not personal failures. They are the predictable outcomes of using the wrong operating system for the mission at hand.

- **The Mission is Evolution, Not Elimination:** The goal is not to kill the powerful predator within you. The goal is to evolve him, transforming his brute force into the precision and control of a master pilot.

- **This is Engineering, Not Magic Tricks:** Forget flimsy tips like "thinking about baseball." We are not applying a band-aid. We are opening the hood of your machine to give you conscious control over the switches that have been running on autopilot.

Chapter 2

The Commander's Intent: Engineering Desire

The Mission Before the Mission

Before a commander sends his troops onto the battlefield, he clarifies one thing above all else: The *Commander's Intent*. This is not a simple objective like "take that hill." It is the core philosophy that defines why that hill must be taken, its place in the bigger picture, and what ultimate success looks like. Is the goal to secure a strategic position, to create a diversion, or to capture a resource? The "what" (take the hill) is meaningless without the "why." When the intent is understood, every soldier on the ground can make the right decisions, even in chaos, even when communication lines are down.

The bedroom is not your battlefield; it is the stage where you conduct your art. But the rule is the same: before you act, you must define the *Intent*.

Your old intent, the one programmed by years of success-driven conditioning, was brutally simple: get to the finish line, fast. The mission was orgasm, and success was measured in speed and intensity. Every completed task in your professional life, every closed deal, every solved problem, has trained your brain to crave one thing above all else: the dopamine hit of *done*. Orgasm provides one of the most powerful hits available. Your nervous system has become ruthlessly efficient at reaching it.

This is the trap hidden inside your success.

Now, it is time to evolve that predator into a commander. The new intent is to shift the entire objective: from a defensive battle against your own anxiety to an offensive mission of engineering a mutual, synchronized experience of pleasure. It is the difference between a frantic sprint and a masterfully paced symphony.

What follows will equip your mental arsenal before we touch a single physical technique, because the real war is won or lost not in your muscles, but in the six inches between your ears. Your body is a loyal soldier; it will execute the mission it is given. It is time to give it a better mission.

The Enemy Within: Performance Anxiety and the Dopamine Trap

The "Why": Your Brain's Reward Conditioning

To defeat the enemy, you must first map the terrain of your own mind. Imagine your brain has two key players in this drama, a pilot and a hijacker on the same plane:

The Commander (Your Prefrontal Cortex): This is the evolved, rational part of your brain sitting right behind your forehead. It is the CEO, the skilled pilot in the cockpit. It sets goals, makes complex plans, and understands long-term strategy. It is the part of you reading this book and nodding in agreement. It desires connection, mutual pleasure, and control.

The Primal Warrior (Your Limbic System): This is the ancient, emotional core of your brain. It is the panicked passenger who thinks the plane is going down. It does not understand quarterly reports or strategic planning. It understands threat, reward, pleasure, and pain. It operates on instinct and craves immediate gratification. Its favorite signal is dopamine, and it will do anything to get its fix.

When your Commander brain codes sex as "the task of reaching orgasm," the entire process becomes focused on that final, powerful dopamine prize. Your Primal Warrior hears this and goes on high alert.

The mission is clear: get the reward. This gives birth to performance anxiety. Your Primal Warrior hijacks the plane, convinced that the only way to avoid a crash is to land as quickly as possible.

You are no longer present and feeling the experience; you are in your head, watching from the outside. You are running a constant, frantic internal checklist: *Am I doing this right? Am I hard enough? Will it be too soon? Is she enjoying it?* Each question is a spike of fear, a jolt of turbulence.

This mental noise, this self-focus, is interpreted by your Primal Warrior as a threat. It sounds the alarm. It triggers the Fight or Flight mode from Chapter 1. Your rational brain loses resources. The Commander loses control to the panicked warrior who just wants to end the *threatening* situation as quickly as possible by reaching the finish line. You have become an observer of your own experience, desperately hoping for a good review.

The "How": The New Strategy

The Commander's Intent is to stage a coup in your own mind. A radical shift in mission objective, a way to calmly retake the cockpit from the hijacker.

Your old, failed mission was: *to have an orgasm and prove my performance.*

Your new, winning mission is: **"to maximize total shared pleasure by focusing on my partner's experience."**

This mental pivot changes the entire dynamic. When you take the focus entirely off your own performance and place it on the external, sensory data of your partner, the rhythm of her breath, the slightest tremor in her skin, the look in her eyes, and the sound she makes when you touch her *just so*, performance anxiety evaporates.

Why? **Because you starve it of its only fuel: self-focus.** The hijacker has nothing to panic about if the flight's objective is no longer about a risky landing but about enjoying the view.

The frantic inner narrator goes quiet. Suddenly, you are not managing a crisis; you are gathering intelligence. Her pleasure becomes your navigation system, your real-time feedback loop.

You are no longer taking an exam; you are on a reconnaissance mission. This shift instantly pulls you out of the panicked Fight or Flight mode and into the calm, controlled state of connection and relaxation: Rest and Digest. Time seems to slow down. Your senses, previously dulled by anxiety, come alive. You are finally flying the plane.

The Sensory Audit Drill: Your First Mental Exercise

This is not a vague idea; it is a trainable skill. This is your first mission to practice this new intent: the *Sensory Audit Drill*.

Objective: For the first five minutes of your next intimate encounter, forbid yourself from thinking about your own pleasure, your erection, or your performance. Your personal outcome is irrelevant for this drill.

Execution: Your sole mission is to conduct a sensory audit. Become a detective of her pleasure. Notice three things you have never noticed before. Is her breathing faster when you touch her neck versus her lower back? Do her hips tilt slightly when you change pressure? Is there a specific word she whispers when she is truly lost in the moment? Notice the tiny details: the way her eyelashes flutter, the change in skin temperature on her shoulders. Your focus is 100% external.

Debrief: After, notice how you felt. Were you in your head, running your checklist? Or were you completely present, reacting to real-time data? Did you feel more or less in control when you were not trying to be in control? This is the first step in rewiring your brain from a performance machine into a pleasure machine.

A Tale of Two Maps: Deconstructing Arousal Arcs

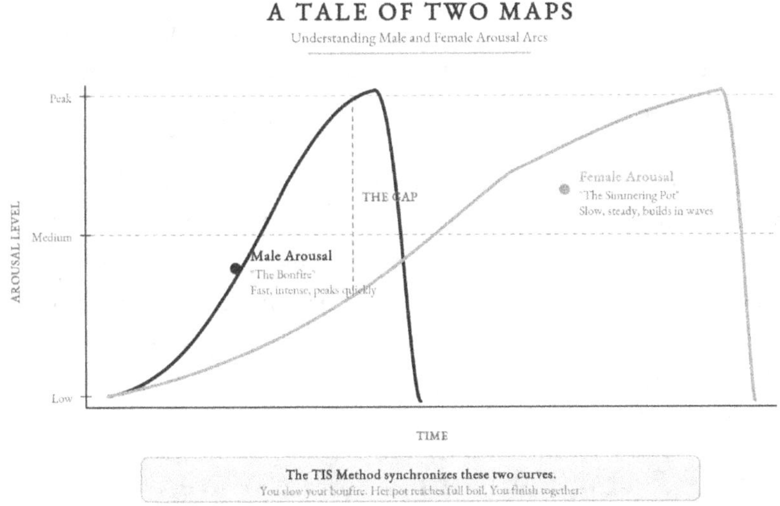

A Tale of Two Maps: Male and Female Arousal Arcs

The "Why": You Have Been Fighting the Terrain

The apex predator mindset makes a fatal error: it assumes the terrain is the same for everyone. It tries to impose its own map on its partner. It is like trying to use a roadmap of a straight desert highway in the middle of a winding mountain range. A commander understands the terrain before he engages.

Men and women, generally speaking, have fundamentally different arousal maps.

The Male Map (The Bonfire): Male arousal is often like building a bonfire. It can be ignited quickly with the right kind of friction, blazes intensely and rapidly to a peak, and after the peak (orgasm), it quickly burns down to embers, often requiring a significant "refractory" period before it can be lit again. It is a powerful, linear, and often swift path. This is a system designed for a single, decisive outcome.

The Female Map (The Simmering Pot): Female arousal is more like bringing a large pot of water to a rolling boil. It requires consistent, steady heat. It builds slowly, reaches a simmer (a plateau), might cool slightly if the heat is removed, and then with sustained attention, climbs to an even more intense boil. Orgasm is often not a single peak, but the highest crest of these waves, and it can be sustained by the momentum of the heat you have already built. Removing the heat source for too long can mean the water cools completely, requiring the process to start over. It is a system designed for a sustained, layered experience.

The predator, with his bonfire roaring, tries to force his partner's pot to boil instantly. He applies intense, direct heat, expecting the same rapid result he experiences. By the time his fire has peaked and is dying down, her water is perhaps just beginning to simmer. This is the moment of complete desynchronization, the source of immense frustration for both partners. He feels like he failed, and she feels like a task that was rushed to completion.

The "How": Pacing Your Climb to Her Waves

The Commander's Intent is to understand these two different maps and to use his fire to patiently heat her water. Your job is not to race to your peak; your job is to become a master of temperature control.

This means a radical re-evaluation of foreplay. For the predator, foreplay is a perfunctory step, a necessary evil before the "main event." For the commander, foreplay is the main event. It is where you build the foundational heat. It is where you observe her map, learn her signals, and begin to synchronize your rhythms. It is the most critical phase of intelligence gathering. It is where you prove through your actions that her pleasure is your priority, building the trust and safety required for her to fully let go.

When you adopt this mindset, "lasting longer" ceases to be a goal you anxiously strive for. It becomes the natural, inevitable consequence of a superior strategy. You last longer because you are no longer in a race against your own body. You are engaged in the far more intricate and rewarding process of stoking her fire and surfing her waves of pleasure.

This chapter is your mental briefing room. The mindset you forge here is the non-negotiable foundation for the physical techniques you will learn in Chapter 3. Remember, the commander sets the intent, and a well-trained body executes that intent flawlessly. When the mind is clear on its mission, the body responds with newfound control and confidence.

Commander's Q&A: Your Mental Operations Briefing

Is focusing on her pleasure not just a different kind of performance anxiety? Now I have to worry about her orgasm!

An excellent and critical question. The key difference is in the nature of the focus. Performance anxiety is rooted in self-judgment (*Am I doing a good job?*). The pleasure-centric mindset is rooted in sensory curiosity (*What is she feeling right now?*). One is an internal interrogation; the other is an external investigation. One creates pressure; the other creates presence. The goal is not to make her orgasm the new "finish line." The goal is to make the exploration of her pleasure the journey itself. Her orgasm becomes a beautiful landmark on a journey you are enjoying together, not the sole destination of a stressful trip.

This sounds great in theory, but what happens when my mind inevitably wanders back to my own sensations and anxieties?

It will. You have years of conditioning to overcome. Do not fight it or judge yourself for it; that only adds another layer of anxiety. Acknowledge the thought, and then gently but firmly pivot your attention back to your mission: the sensory audit. Think of it like a trained soldier hearing a distracting noise. He does not panic; he acknowledges the sound, assesses it as non-threatening, and returns his focus to his objective. A practical way to do this is to change what you are doing with your hands or mouth. This physical shift helps create a mental one.

This whole "Commander's Intent" feels a bit clinical and unromantic. Where is the spontaneity?

Think of a world-class dancer. When he performs on stage, it looks effortless, completely spontaneous. That effortlessness is the product of ten thousand hours of rehearsing positions, learning choreography, and building muscle memory until the technique disappears into the art. Right now, your "spontaneity" is likely dictated by your anxiety, which is the opposite of freedom. By mastering your internal state with this new intent, you create the mental and emotional freedom for true, authentic spontaneity to emerge. You are learning the steps so you can eventually lose yourself in the dance.

Why is this mental shift so important to do before learning the physical techniques?

Because if you learn the physical techniques in Chapter 3 with the old "predator" mindset, you will simply turn them into more efficient weapons for racing to the finish line. You will use the breath control to push yourself harder, not to relax. You will use the rhythm control to create more intensity, not to manage it. The physical tools are only as effective as the intent of the man who wields them. A hammer can be used to build a house or to demolish it; the tool is the same, but the intent changes everything. Mindset first. Always.

Commander's Briefing: Chapter 2

- **The Commander's Intent Defines the Mission:** Before a commander engages, he defines why and what success looks like. Your new intent shifts the objective from "prove my performance" to "maximize total shared pleasure by focusing on my partner's experience."

- **You Are Piloting a Hijacked Plane:** Your mind has two operators: The calm, strategic Commander (your rational brain) and the panicked, instinct-driven Primal Warrior (your emotional brain). When the mission is "performance," the Primal Warrior hijacks the controls and initiates an emergency landing.

- **Starve the Enemy of its Fuel:** Performance anxiety feeds on one thing: self-focus. By shifting your entire attention outward, to the sensory data of her pleasure (her breath, her touch, her sounds), you cut off anxiety's only supply line. The hijacker is neutralized because the "threat" has vanished.

- **You Have Been Using the Wrong Map:** Male arousal is a bonfire (fast, intense, peaks quickly). Female arousal is a simmering pot (slow, steady heat, builds in waves). Trying to force her pot to boil with your bonfire is a guaranteed mission failure.

- **Foreplay is the Main Event:** For the predator, foreplay was a preliminary step. For the commander, foreplay is the battlefield. It is where you gather intelligence, build foundational heat, and synchronize your rhythms. Lasting longer is not the goal; it is the inevitable consequence of a superior strategy.

- **The Mind Must Be Conquered Before the Body Can Be Commanded:** This mindset is the non-negotiable foundation for the physical techniques in Chapter 3. Without the right intent, even the best technique becomes a weapon for racing to the finish line.

THE SYNCHRONIZATION ENGINE: TACTICS FOR TOTAL CONTROL

Three Men, One Secret

JOHN IS A 28-YEAR-OLD software engineer. He ships features under impossible deadlines, debugs million-line codebases, and has earned the nickname "the machine" for his unflappable focus. His team sees him as unshakeable.

At home, with his girlfriend, he is anything but.

They had been together for two years. Good years, mostly. She was patient, understanding, the kind of woman who said "it's okay" and seemed to mean it. But John had started to notice things. The way her "it's okay" came a little too quickly now, almost rehearsed. The way she had stopped initiating. The way she scrolled her phone in bed afterward, filling the silence with something, anything.

Two minutes. Sometimes three on a good night. That was his window. Two years of trying to extend it, two years of mental gymnastics and breathing exercises and "think about something else." Nothing worked. Not reliably. Not when it mattered.

The worst part was the anticipation. In the hours before they would be intimate, John felt the anxiety building. Not excitement. Dread. The familiar loop: *Maybe tonight will be different. But it won't be. And she'll say it's okay. And we'll both know it isn't.*

He had started making excuses. "Long day." "Early meeting tomorrow." "Not feeling great." Anything to avoid the encounter that reminded him of his inadequacy.

One night, lying in the dark after another abbreviated session, she whispered: "John, are we okay?"

He knew what she was really asking. And he did not have an answer.

"We're fine," he said.

The lie sat between them like a third person in the bed.

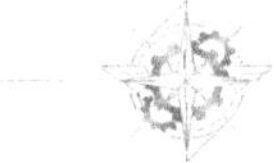

Matt is a 38-year-old trauma surgeon. He holds beating hearts in his hands. He makes split-second decisions that determine whether someone walks out of the hospital or gets wheeled to the morgue. In the operating theater, his hands never tremble.

In bed with his wife, those same hands shake with performance anxiety.

It had not always been this way. When they first married, before the residency hours and the overnight calls and the bone-deep exhaustion, things were different. Spontaneous. Passionate. His wife used to joke that they were making up for lost time whenever they were together.

Now, eight years and one child later, intimacy had become a scheduled event. Wednesday nights if they were lucky, after their son was asleep, in the narrow window before Matt's body surrendered to fatigue. And in that precious window, the same pattern repeated: connection attempted, connection shortened, connection abandoned.

"It's the stress," his wife would say, being generous. "The hospital. Everything you carry."

She was not wrong. But she was not entirely right either.

Matt had performed surgeries for fourteen hours straight without his hands trembling. He had delivered death notifications to families with composure and grace. He had earned a reputation for being unshakeable in the most extreme circumstances medicine could offer.

Why, then, could he not maintain control in his own bedroom?

His eight-year-old son had asked a question recently that cut deeper than any scalpel. They were at the playground, just the two of them, a rare afternoon off.

"Daddy," his son said, watching a couple hold hands across the park, "why doesn't Mommy look at you like that lady looks at that man?"

Matt did not have an answer. He deflected, pointed at the swings, changed the subject.

That night, he watched his wife across the dinner table. His son was right. There was a flatness in her eyes when she looked at him now. Not anger. Not resentment. Something worse: resignation.

He was a surgeon. He fixed things. He saved lives.

Why couldn't he save this?

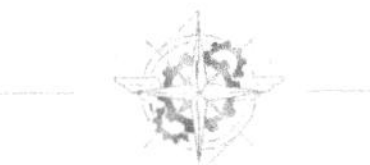

David is a 41-year-old construction project manager. He coordinates two hundred workers across multiple sites. He juggles million-dollar timelines and solves crises before his morning coffee gets cold. On the job site, he is unshakable.

In the bedroom, after fifteen years of marriage, he had no idea he was failing.

That is the thing about David. He thought he was normal. One minute, maybe two on a good night. That was just how it worked, right? Every guy finished fast. The movies exaggerated. His buddies at poker night sure as hell were not bragging about marathon sessions.

Then came the joke.

They were lying in bed after another sixty-second encounter. His wife stared at the ceiling, that familiar silence filling the room. Then she turned to him with a half-smile.

"You know," she said, "for that, I probably didn't need to take off my pants."

She laughed. He laughed too, reflexively. But something cracked open in that moment.

She was not being cruel. That was her way, always had been. Humor instead of confrontation. But the message landed like a construction beam to the chest: This is not enough. This has never been enough. And you didn't even know.

David spent the next week in a quiet crisis. He started paying attention, something he had avoided for fifteen years. He noticed her face after they finished, the way her smile never quite reached her eyes. He noticed she had stopped initiating months ago. Maybe years. He noticed the distance that had grown between their bodies in sleep, the six inches of mattress that might as well have been a canyon.

"All this time," he told his reflection one morning, shaving for work, "I thought I was fine. I thought we were fine."

They were not fine. But David was about to learn that the gap between where he was and where he needed to be was smaller than he feared. Closeable. Trainable. Mechanical.

His wife's joke became the best gift she ever gave him.

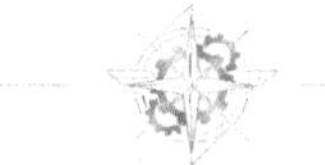

John, Matt, and David are not outliers. They are the norm. And if you see yourself in any of them, whether you command a boardroom, an operating theater, a construction site, a classroom, a kitchen, or a delivery truck, you are exactly where you need to be.

This chapter is where theory becomes practice. You have learned why your body betrays you. You have adopted the Commander's Intent. Now it is time to build the engine that will give you control. Not the illusion of control. Real, mechanical, repeatable control.

I call it the *Synchronization Engine*: three integrated tactics that work together like pistons in a motor. Each tactic serves a specific function. Together, they synchronize your control mechanisms with your partner's arousal, creating an experience neither of you will forget.

This is the heart of the TIS Method. Let us begin.

The Three Tactics

Your tactical overview before we proceed:

Tactic 1: *The Reset* The pre-fatigue bio-hack that disarms your ejaculatory reflex before you even begin. This is your foundation. Your non-negotiable.

Tactic 2: *The Breath* The coherence breathing pattern that keeps your nervous system calm during penetration. This amplifies your control.

Tactic 3: *The Rhythm* The wave synchronization technique that transforms mechanical sex into an art form. This is where mastery lives.

One of these tactics is mandatory. The other two are force multipliers. By the end of this chapter, you will understand why, and you will know exactly how to execute each one.

Let us begin with the one that changes everything.

Tactic 1: The Reset (The Pre-Fatigue Bio-Hack)

The Discovery

Marriage, I learned early, is not a destination. It is a craft.

I grew up watching the marriages around me. Some deepened over decades, the couples still reaching for each other's hands at holiday dinners. Others slowly hollowed out, the husbands and wives sitting at opposite ends of the table with nothing left to say. The difference fascinated me.

A family friend, married fifty-three years, pulled me aside at a wedding once and said something I never forgot: "Son, a happy wife is not an accident. It is a daily practice. And most of that practice happens behind closed doors."

When I married my wife, I made a decision: I would not leave the quality of our relationship to chance. I turned to the research, and what I found confirmed what that older generation understood intuitively. When your partner consistently reaches completion, her biochemistry transforms. Oxytocin floods her system, strengthening neurological bonds with each encounter. Cortisol drops. Anxiety recedes. She becomes more patient, more affectionate, more deeply connected to her partner.

And when she does not? Distance grows. Resentment builds, often unconsciously. She may not articulate why she feels disconnected, but her nervous system knows. No amount of gifts or date nights can substitute for what is missing.

Sexual satisfaction is not a luxury in a marriage. It is foundational architecture.

But I faced the same challenge most men face: biology. Most women require sustained stimulation to reach orgasm, often fifteen to twenty minutes or more. Most men, left to their natural reflexes, finish far sooner. This is not a character flaw. It is physiology. The ejaculatory reflex evolved for reproduction, not for mutual pleasure.

Could that physiology be trained?

I tried the obvious approaches first. Mental distraction felt like betrayal: how could I be fully present with my wife while calculating numbers? Numbing creams stole sensation from both of us. The stop-start method broke our rhythm and her building arousal. Each "technique" solved one problem while creating another.

The deeper I researched, the more I understood the core challenge. Every approach assumed you could consciously override an unconscious reflex in the heat of the moment. But the ejaculatory reflex is controlled by the autonomic nervous system, the same system that governs heartbeat and pupil dilation. You cannot will it not to fire any more than you can will yourself not to blink.

I needed a fundamentally different approach.

Around this time, I had been doing pelvic floor exercises. Strengthening exercises showed clear results: stronger contractions, more intense sensations. But reverse Kegels during arousal were nearly impossible. The moment stimulation intensified, the muscle contracted despite my efforts. I was trying to relax a spring that was determined to snap.

Then came the breakthrough.

During a strengthening session, I held a maximum contraction longer than usual. Twenty seconds, perhaps twenty-five, pushing the muscle to complete fatigue. When I finally released, I noticed something unexpected.

The muscle felt empty. Depleted. Exhausted.

Curious, I touched myself experimentally. Normally, any contact with sensitive areas triggered an immediate reflexive clench. This time: nothing. The muscle was too tired to respond.

And critically, I was still fully erect.

The anatomy made sense when I thought it through. Erection is hydraulic: blood flows into the corpus cavernosum and is trapped there. Ejaculation is muscular: the pelvic floor contracts rhythmically to expel semen. These are separate systems. Fatiguing the muscle does not release the blood. You remain aroused. You simply lose the hair-trigger reflex that ends things prematurely.

I had spent months trying to relax a muscle that refused to relax. The answer was not relaxation.

The answer was exhaustion.

That night, I tried it with my wife. During foreplay, I discreetly held a maximum pelvic contraction for twenty seconds, then released. When we proceeded, the difference was immediate. The familiar urgency was absent. I felt pleasure without panic. Arousal without the racing countdown.

When stimulation eventually built toward the threshold, I withdrew briefly, executed another contraction hold, and returned with my control restored.

For the first time, I chose when we finished. Together.

In the weeks that followed, I refined the technique. I discovered that my control window lengthened as my pelvic floor grew stronger. I learned that coherence breathing could extend the intervals between resets. I experimented with penetration rhythms that optimized stimulation for both of us.

And I watched my marriage transform.

My wife became more affectionate. More patient. More at peace. She reached for my hand more often. She looked at me the way she had in our earliest days. The bedroom was transforming everything outside of it.

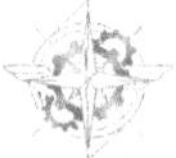

Eventually, I shared the technique with three men I trusted.

John was my neighbor, a 28-year-old software engineer who lived two doors down. We had become friends over backyard barbecues and borrowed tools. One evening, after a few beers on his patio, he confided something he had never told anyone. At 28, he should have been at his peak. Instead, he dreaded intimacy with his girlfriend.

Matt was a father I had met through our kids' school. Our sons were in the same class, and we had bonded over countless basketball games and school pickups. He was a trauma surgeon, a man who held beating hearts in his hands, yet one afternoon in the parking lot, he admitted his marriage was straining under the weight of unspoken disappointment.

David was my oldest friend, someone I had known for over a decade. At 41, married for fifteen years, he had recently heard a joke from his wife that cracked something open in him. He called me the next day, shaken. "I think I've been failing her," he said. "For years. And I just realized it."

I gave each of them the same system you now hold in your hands. I asked them to practice it seriously, to involve their partners, and to report back honestly.

Every one of them came back with the same message.

"It works. Every time. I cannot believe how simple it is."

"My wife asked what changed. She said it feels like dating again."

"I feel like I have a superpower. Like I can control anything now."

Their transformations convinced me that this system needed to be shared more widely. Their stories, which you will follow throughout this book, are the proof that what I discovered is not a fluke. It is replicable, teachable, and life-changing.

You will meet John, Matt, and David again in other chapters. You will see their struggles and their victories. By the end, their success will feel inevitable.

And so will yours.

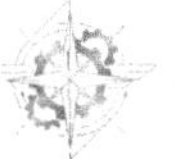

That sense of control radiates outward. The confidence that comes from mastering this challenge does not stay in the bedroom. It bleeds into work, fitness, relationships, every domain of life. When you prove to yourself that you can control your body's most primal reflex, everything else feels manageable.

This book is my attempt to give that same experience to every man who wants it. The technique you are about to learn, The Reset, is not theoretical. It has been tested, refined, validated by others, and grounded in muscle physiology that any doctor would recognize.

You are not broken. You are not uniquely disadvantaged. You have simply not been given the right tool.

Now you have it.

The Science

Your *bulbospongiosus* and *ischiocavernosus* muscles, the pelvic floor muscles responsible for triggering ejaculation, operate like any other muscle. When you push them to maximum contraction and hold, they enter a refractory state. They literally cannot fire at full strength again until they recover.

This is the same reason your biceps cannot lift another heavy weight immediately after a maximum effort set. The muscle needs recovery time. During this recovery window, it can only achieve partial contraction, well below its full capacity. The critical insight: partial contraction is below the threshold required to trigger the ejaculatory reflex.

You are not fighting your reflex. You are preemptively disarming it.

Identifying Your Pelvic Floor

If you are unfamiliar with pelvic floor exercises (often called Kegels), the contraction is the same motion you would use to stop urination midstream. This is your target muscle group.

To verify you have identified the correct muscles, try this during urination: start the flow, then stop it completely. The muscles you use to halt the stream are your pelvic floor muscles. These are the muscles you will contract during The Reset.

Important: Do not practice Resets by actually stopping urination. This can lead to incomplete bladder emptying and potential urinary issues. Use this only as a one-time identification exercise.

Once you have identified the sensation, you can practice contractions anytime: sitting at your desk, driving, or during dedicated training sessions. For a comprehensive eight-week training protocol, see Appendix E: Pelvic Floor Training Fundamentals.

The Execution

Timing: During foreplay, before penetration begins. Your partner does not need to know what you are doing. You are simply... focusing.

The Protocol:

Contract your pelvic floor as strongly as you possibly can. Imagine you are stopping urination midstream, but harder. Maximum effort. A critical note: you are contracting the internal muscles, not your glutes, thighs, or abdominals. If you notice your buttocks clenching, your legs tensing, or your abdomen tightening, you are recruiting the wrong muscles. The correct contraction should feel deep and internal, centered between your sit bones. Your outer body should remain relatively still while the internal squeeze is at maximum. If you are unsure, practice in front of a mirror. When done correctly, there should be minimal visible movement.

Hold this contraction for fifteen to twenty seconds. Your muscles will begin to fatigue. You may feel a burning sensation, a slight tremble, or simply a growing difficulty in maintaining the contraction. Any of these signals indicate you are approaching the fatigue threshold. This is what we want.

Release. Do not try to keep the muscle relaxed. Do not think about it at all. Simply let go.

Proceed to penetration within the next thirty seconds, while the muscle is still fatigued.

What You Will Feel:

When you enter your partner, you will notice something remarkable. That familiar reflexive clench? Absent. You will feel sensation, but your pelvic floor will remain at low tension, a fraction of its usual reactivity. You are in control. Not because you are fighting anything, but because the fight has been preemptively won.

The Reset During Intercourse

This is where the tactic becomes truly powerful.

You will reach a point during intercourse where, despite starting from a fatigued state, arousal builds and the ejaculatory reflex begins to assert itself. You will feel it coming. This is normal.

When this happens:

Withdraw from your partner. Smoothly. Confidently. This is not retreat; it is tactical repositioning.

Immediately contract your pelvic floor at maximum effort again. Hold for twelve to fifteen seconds.

During this hold, continue foreplay. Kiss her. Touch her. Whisper to her. She stays engaged; you are resetting your system.

You will feel the ejaculatory pressure dissipate. It is almost like the sensation retreats downward, away from the *Point of No Return*.

Re-enter when you feel the reset complete.

I have used this technique to extend intimate sessions indefinitely. Each reset buys you another extended window of control. And something interesting happens: the pleasure does not diminish with each reset. It compounds. By the time you choose to finish, the intensity is extraordinary.

The Mental Amplifier

This technique works on a purely physical level. Muscle fatigue is muscle fatigue, regardless of your mental state. But your mindset can dramatically amplify or diminish its effectiveness.

When the ejaculatory sensation begins to build and you withdraw to execute a Reset, you face a choice. You can think: *This is hopeless. I am going to finish anyway. Why bother holding?* This thought triggers anxiety, spikes your sympathetic nervous system, and works against the Reset.

Or you can think: *I am in control. I can hold this. Every second I hold, the sensation retreats further. When I return, I will have even more control than before.* This thought maintains your parasympathetic state and allows the Reset to work optimally.

Every time you successfully execute a Reset, every time you prove to yourself that you can hold, you build something more valuable than technique. You build confidence. You build identity. You become the man who chooses when to finish.

Your partner will feel the difference. Not the technique itself, but the result. A man who can extend pleasure indefinitely, who can read her responses and adjust, who can bring her to peaks she did not know existed. That man stands apart. Not because of size. Not because of some genetic gift. Because of function. Because of what he can do. The one she cannot stop thinking about. The one who makes her feel truly seen and satisfied.

A word of caution: this is not about marathon sessions for their own sake. Extended intimacy should serve mutual pleasure, not your ego. Learn to read when your partner is satisfied, when she craves the crescendo. The goal is shared ecstasy, not endurance records. There is a point where more becomes too much, and wisdom lies in recognizing it. But when you have the ability to extend, you also have the ability to choose the perfect moment to finish together. That choice is the ultimate gift you can offer.

Plant this seed in your mind: *I can hold. I choose when we finish. This is my gift to both of us.*

Individual Variation and the Power of Progressive Training

Your optimal Reset hold time depends on your current pelvic floor strength. This is your starting point, not your ceiling.

If you have never trained these muscles, you might achieve fatigue in ten seconds. A weaker pelvic floor means shorter control windows between Resets. You may need to execute multiple Resets during a single encounter initially. This is normal. This is expected. And this will change.

The Science of Strength

Your pelvic floor muscles, the bulbospongiosus and ischiocavernosus, follow the same physiological principles as your biceps, your quadriceps, or any other skeletal muscle in your body. When you subject a muscle to progressive resistance training, three adaptations occur:

First, neural efficiency increases. Your brain learns to recruit more muscle fibers simultaneously, generating stronger contractions with the same tissue. This happens within the first two to four weeks of consistent training.

Second, muscle fiber hypertrophy begins. The individual fibers thicken, increasing their force-generating capacity. This becomes measurable after six to eight weeks of regular exercise.

Third, fatigue resistance improves. Trained muscles develop enhanced capillary networks and mitochondrial density, allowing them to sustain contractions longer before exhaustion. This is the adaptation that transforms your Reset from a temporary pause into a decisive weapon.

The implication is profound: the same Reset technique becomes exponentially more powerful as your foundation strengthens.

The Levels of Mastery

Think of pelvic floor development in four stages:

Level 1 — Beginner: Your Reset provides a brief window of control. You may need three, four, even five Resets during a single intimate session. Each Reset buys you enough time to continue, but the intervals feel short. This is where most men start.

Level 2 — Developing: Your Reset provides a meaningful control window. Two or three Resets per session become sufficient. You begin to relax into the rhythm of intimate connection rather than constantly monitoring your state.

Level 3 — Proficient: A single Reset at the beginning, combined with The Breath and The Rhythm, carries you through an entire encounter. You Reset mid-session only by choice, not necessity. Your partner notices the difference. You have become the exception.

Level 4 — Master: The initial pre-penetration Reset, executed as second nature, provides complete control for as long as you choose. You decide when the encounter ends. The ejaculatory reflex has become fully subordinate to your intention. This is the level where intimacy transforms from performance into art.

The distance between Level 1 and Level 4 is not talent. It is training.

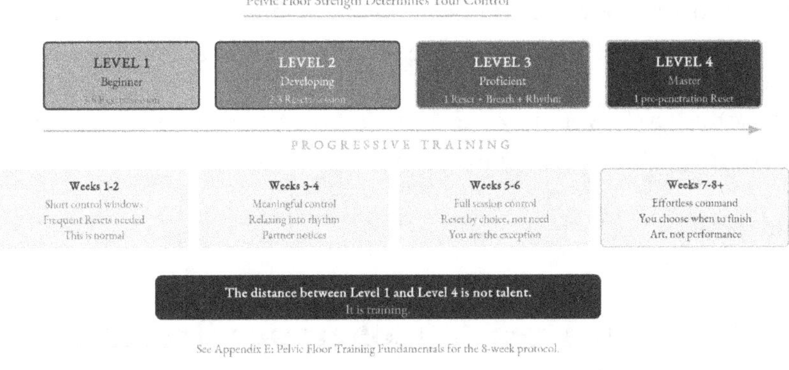

The Four Levels of Mastery

Your Training Resources

Building this foundation requires consistent, progressive exercise. You have multiple pathways available:

The Pelvic Floor Training Fundamentals appendix at the end of this book provides a complete eight-week protocol you can follow immediately, no equipment or technology required.

See Appendix E: Pelvic Floor Training Fundamentals for the complete protocol, or visit tismethod.com/tactical-intimacy/book-owners for digital training tools including adaptive progression and real-time guidance.

Choose the method that fits your life. The key is consistency, not complexity. Ten minutes of daily practice, sustained over weeks, will carry you from Level 1 toward Level 4 more reliably than any amount of sporadic effort.

The Non-Negotiable Truth

Do not skip this training.

The Reset technique works from day one, even with an untrained pelvic floor. You will experience improvement tonight if you apply what you have learned. But the men who achieve true mastery, the ones who reach Level 4, are the ones who invest in the foundation.

Your pelvic floor is the engine of this entire system. A stronger engine means longer control windows, fewer interruptions, deeper presence, and ultimately, the ability to orchestrate intimate experiences that your partner will never forget.

Your starting level is your baseline. Level 4 is your destination. The path between them is paved with consistent daily practice.

Begin today.

Tactic 2: The Breath (Coherence Breathing)

The Foundation

Once you have executed The Reset and penetration has begun, you need a way to maintain your parasympathetic state. You need to keep your nervous system from tipping back into Fight or Flight mode. This is where breath becomes your anchor.

James Nestor, the journalist and author who wrote *Breath: The New Science of a Lost Art*, documented a fascinating finding. Researchers studying prayer, meditation, and traditional breathing practices across cultures discovered they all converged on the same rhythm: approximately 5.5 seconds inhale, 5.5 seconds exhale. This is not coincidence. This rhythm, roughly five to six breaths per minute, triggers what scientists call *respiratory sinus arrhythmia* and maximizes

Heart Rate Variability.

Heart Rate Variability, or *HRV*, measures your nervous system's flexibility. A healthy heart does not beat like a metronome; it speeds up slightly on inhale and slows down on exhale. High HRV indicates parasympathetic dominance, the Rest and Digest state where ejaculatory control lives. (For a detailed explanation of HRV and its role in sexual function, see the Glossary.)

The Practical Problem

Now, you might be thinking: *How am I supposed to count 5.5 seconds while I am having sex?*

You are not. The method is straightforward:

Forget the half-second. Think of it as a slow five-count. In your mind, count "one… two… three… four… five" at a relaxed pace as you inhale. Then the same count as you exhale. You are not aiming for stopwatch precision. You are aiming for a slow, deliberate rhythm that prevents the rapid, shallow breathing that accompanies arousal and anxiety.

The goal is approximately five to six complete breath cycles per minute. If you are anywhere in that range, you are in coherence.

The Execution

When to Begin: Start this breathing pattern as penetration begins, right after you have executed The Reset. This becomes your background operating system for the entire encounter.

The Pattern:

Inhale slowly through your nose for a count of five

Exhale slowly through your nose for a count of five

Maintain this rhythm continuously during intercourse

What You Will Notice:

Your heart rate will stabilize. The frantic, pounding sensation that accompanies high arousal will soften into something more controlled. Time will seem to dilate slightly. You will feel more present, more aware of your partner, less trapped in your own anxious thoughts.

Combining With Tactic 1

When you feel arousal building toward the danger zone, you have two tools working together. Your pre-fatigued pelvic floor provides the physical buffer. Your *Coherence Breathing* keeps your nervous system from amplifying the signals. Together, they extend your control window dramatically.

And when you need to execute a Reset, the breath gives you something to focus on during those fifteen seconds. Inhale, hold the pelvic contraction, exhale, maintain the hold. The breathing pattern keeps you calm and present while the muscle fatigues.

A Note on Erection Concerns

Some men worry that calming down will cost them their erection. This is a valid concern if you are using breath alone, outside of sexual activity. Deep relaxation can indeed reduce arousal.

The reason it works during penetration: you have constant physical stimulation maintaining arousal. The breath is not eliminating arousal; it is preventing arousal from spiking into the panic zone. You are not trying to calm down to zero. You are trying to stay in the optimal window: aroused enough to maintain erection, calm enough to maintain control.

The combination of physical stimulation plus coherence breathing creates the perfect balance. Relaxed alertness. Controlled arousal. This is the state where you can last as long as you choose.

For the Breath Pacer and guided coherence breathing tools, visit tismethod.com/tactical-intimacy/book-owners or see Appendix A: TIS Digital Resources for registration details.

Tactic 3: The Rhythm (Wave Synchronization)

The Ancient Wisdom

The Taoists understood something about sexual dynamics that modern men have largely forgotten. They developed penetration rhythms that balance stimulation, prevent desensitization, and synchronize the arousal curves of both partners. The most widely known ratio: nine shallow strokes, then one deep stroke. Repeat.

Some practitioners prefer simpler variations. Three shallow, one deep. Five shallow, one deep. The exact ratio matters less than the principle: predominantly shallow, occasionally deep. The rhythm should feel natural, not mathematical. Find what works for you and your partner.

This is not mystical nonsense. It is biomechanical wisdom.

Why It Works

For You:

The most sensitive part of the penis is the glans, the head. During shallow strokes, the glans remains near the entrance of the vagina, where nerve endings are less densely stimulated than in full penetration. You receive pleasure, but at a lower intensity that is easier to control.

The single deep stroke provides a spike of intense sensation, the full-depth pleasure that your body craves, but it is brief. Before that intensity can accumulate and push you toward the threshold, you return to the lower-intensity shallow strokes.

You are essentially cycling between *recovery* and *intensity* phases, giving your nervous system constant micro-breaks without sacrificing the experience.

For Your Partner:

Women typically have significant nerve endings in the outer third of the vaginal canal. Shallow strokes stimulate this region repeatedly. The single deep stroke stimulates the deeper areas, including the potential for cervical contact, which many women find intensely pleasurable.

More importantly, this varied rhythm creates waves of sensation rather than monotonous friction. It builds anticipation. She never knows exactly when that deep stroke is coming. This psychological element amplifies her physical arousal.

Defining "Shallow" and "Deep"

This requires individual calibration. There is no universal percentage.

A shallow stroke might be fifty percent penetration for one couple and seventy percent for another, depending on anatomy, position, and comfort. The key is not hitting a specific depth; the key is maintaining relaxed, unhurried movement.

A wise warning: during deep strokes, do not *power through*. Many men unconsciously tense their entire lower body when attempting full penetration, engaging glutes, core, and crucially, the pelvic floor. This is the opposite of what we want. A deep stroke should be a smooth glide, not a forceful thrust. Your hips move forward, your pelvic floor stays as relaxed as possible.

If you find yourself tensing to achieve depth, you are pushing too hard. Ease back. Let the depth come naturally from hip movement, not from muscular force. The purpose of the deep stroke is not to demonstrate power; it is to provide variety. Both you and your partner benefit from the change in sensation, not from the force behind it.

The Execution

Starting the Pattern:

After executing The Reset and beginning penetration with coherence breathing established, introduce the rhythm gradually. Start with five shallow, one deep. As you settle into the pattern, extend to nine shallow, one deep.

Counting Without Obsessing:

You do not need to count precisely every time. The ratio matters less than the principle. Mostly shallow, occasionally deep. If you lose count, that is fine. The point is to avoid the reflexive *piston* motion where every stroke is at maximum depth and maximum speed.

Reading Your Partner:

Watch her responses. Some women prefer more deep strokes. Some prefer more shallow. The Taoist ratio is a starting framework, not a rigid law. Adjust based on what you observe in her breathing, her movements, her sounds. This is where the art of Tactic 3 lives.

The Synchronization Effect

When all three tactics combine, something remarkable happens. Your pre-fatigued pelvic floor removes the hair-trigger reflex. Your coherence breathing keeps your nervous system calm. Your varied rhythm prevents stimulation from accumulating too rapidly.

While you are managing your arousal, the rhythm is building hers. The varied tempo, the anticipation, the extended duration, these elements combine to create an experience that is profoundly satisfying for both partners.

You are not just lasting longer. You are conducting a symphony. Two arousal curves, once hopelessly out of sync, now rising together toward a shared crescendo.

This is the Synchronization Engine in full operation.

Assembling the Engine: Your Pre-Flight Checklist

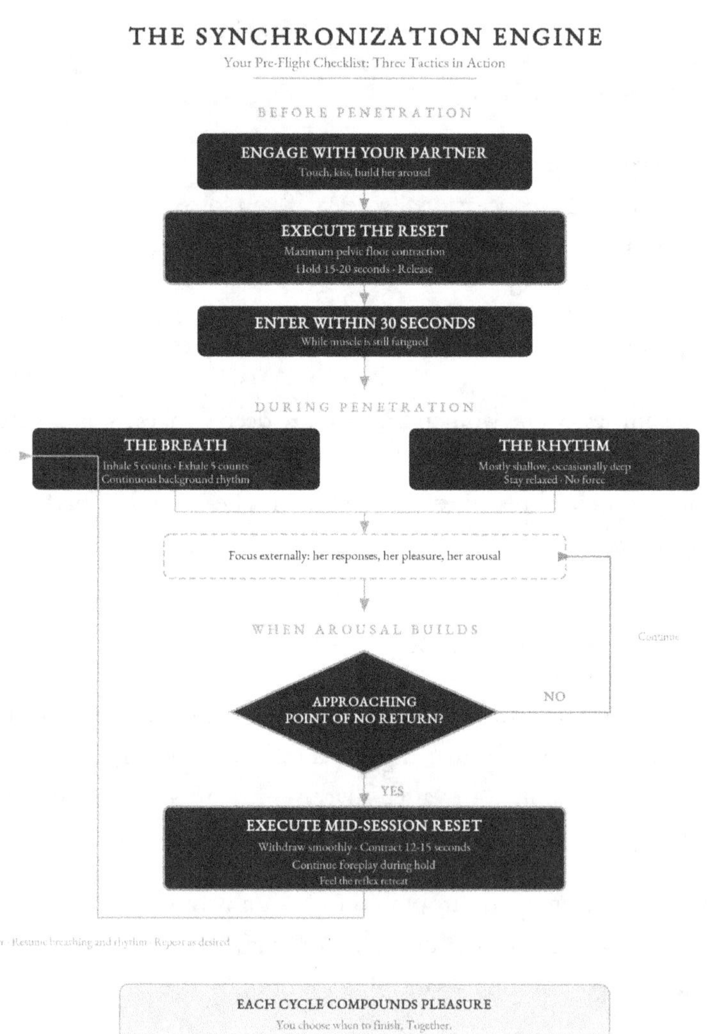

The Synchronization Engine: Pre-Flight Checklist

Let me walk you through how these three tactics integrate into a single, seamless system.

Before Penetration (Foreplay Phase):

Engage with your partner fully. Touch, kiss, build her arousal.

At some point before you intend to penetrate, discreetly execute Tactic 1: The Reset. Contract your pelvic floor maximally for 15-20 seconds. She does not need to know.

Allow the muscle to release. You now have a window of suppressed reflex response.

During Penetration:

As you enter, begin Tactic 2: The Breath. Slow inhale for five counts, slow exhale for five counts. This becomes your background rhythm.

Introduce Tactic 3: The Rhythm. Mostly shallow strokes, occasional deep strokes. Stay relaxed. No forceful thrusting.

Focus externally on her responses, her pleasure, her arousal building. This is the Commander's Intent from Chapter 2 in action.

When Arousal Builds:

You will feel the ejaculatory sensation begin to rise despite your tactics. This is normal.

Before reaching the Point of No Return, withdraw smoothly.

Execute another Reset. Fifteen seconds, maximum contraction.

During the hold, maintain engagement with her. Foreplay continues.

When the Reset completes and the sensation retreats, re-enter.

Resume breathing and rhythm.

Repeat as desired.

Each cycle buys you another extended window. The compound effect of multiple controlled approaches creates an intensity of final release that is difficult to describe. You have to experience it.

The TIS Tactical Hierarchy

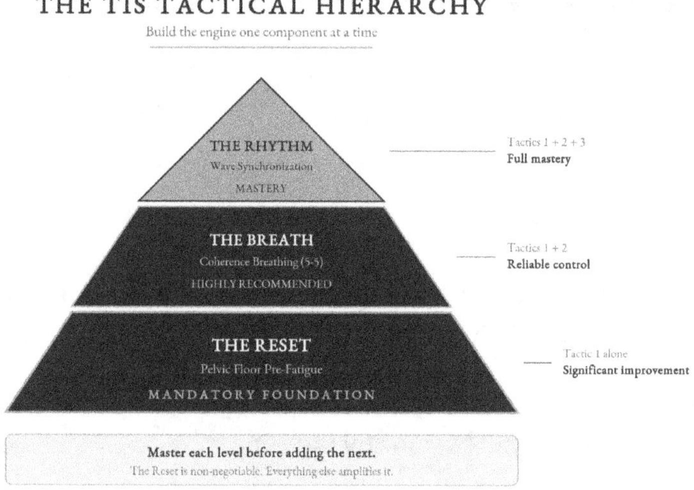

The TIS Tactical Hierarchy

Now that you understand all three tactics, let me be direct about their relative importance.

Tactic 1: The Reset — MANDATORY

This is your foundation. Without pre-fatiguing your pelvic floor, you are fighting an uphill battle against an unconscious reflex. You might achieve control through willpower alone, but it will be inconsistent and exhausting. The Reset removes the reflex from the equation. Everything else builds on this.

Tactic 2: The Breath — HIGHLY RECOMMENDED

Coherence breathing amplifies your control significantly. It keeps your nervous system from spiking into panic mode. It extends the intervals between Resets. However, if for some reason you cannot maintain the breathing pattern, The Reset alone will still give you meaningful control. You will simply need to Reset more frequently.

Tactic 3: The Rhythm — RECOMMENDED FOR MASTERY

The shallow-deep pattern is the difference between mere endurance and true artistry. It optimizes pleasure for both partners and creates the synchronization effect that transforms sex from an anxious performance into a shared experience. However, again, if you struggle with the rhythm, Tactics 1 and 2 alone will still dramatically improve your control.

The Hierarchy:

Tactic 1 alone: Significant improvement over no system

Tactics 1 + 2: Major improvement, reliable control

Tactics 1 + 2 + 3: Full mastery, transformative experience

Start with mastering The Reset. Add The Breath when The Reset becomes automatic. Add The Rhythm when the first two are integrated. Do not try to implement all three simultaneously on your first attempt. Build the engine one component at a time.

Commander's Q&A: Your Tactical Operations Briefing

What if I cannot hold the pelvic contraction for twenty seconds? My muscle gives out earlier.

Then hold for as long as you can. If your maximum is ten seconds, that is your current threshold. The fatigue principle still applies. You will simply have shorter control windows and may need to Reset more frequently. Over time, as you practice pelvic floor strengthening, your endurance will increase, and your Reset duration will extend. The eight-week progressive protocol in Appendix E: Pelvic Floor Training Fundamentals will build your strength systematically.

Is it not obvious to my partner that I am doing something when I contract my pelvic floor for twenty seconds?

Not if you do it during foreplay. She is engaged with what you are doing to her. Your internal muscle contraction is invisible. You might hold your breath slightly or focus your gaze, but these are easily attributed to arousal. Most partners will never notice.

What if I withdraw for a Reset and my erection starts to fade?

This is where maintaining foreplay during the Reset is critical. Keep stimulation going. Touch her, kiss her, whisper to her. The brief withdrawal combined with continued engagement typically maintains arousal for both of you. If you find erection fading, reduce the Reset hold time slightly and ensure you are re-entering promptly once the ejaculatory pressure subsides.

How do I know when my Reset is "complete"? When is it safe to re-enter?

You will feel the ejaculatory pressure dissipate. Many men describe it as the sensation "retreating" or "dropping back." The urgent feeling of imminent release fades into general arousal. This typically happens around the ten to fifteen second mark of your hold, sometimes earlier if you caught the sensation early. With practice, you will recognize this shift clearly.

The 9:1 rhythm feels mechanical and takes me out of the moment. Any advice?

Stop counting precisely. The ratio is a guideline, not a prescription. Think of it as "mostly shallow, occasionally deep." Let it become intuitive rather than mathematical. Focus on what feels good and what generates response from your partner. The principle matters more than the exact count.

Do I have to use all three tactics every time, or can I just use The Reset?

You can absolutely rely on The Reset alone, especially while you are learning. Many men find that Tactic 1 alone gives them the control they need. Add the other tactics as you become more comfortable and want to refine your experience. There is no requirement to implement everything at once.

I have been doing Kegels for years. Will the Reset still work for me?

Yes, but you may need longer hold times to achieve fatigue. A highly trained pelvic floor is stronger but still subject to the same fatigue principles. Experiment with holds of twenty-five to thirty seconds. Find the duration that creates the "no reflex" window for you.

One important exception: if years of Kegels have left you with pelvic tension, discomfort, or trouble fully relaxing the muscle, more contraction is NOT the answer. You may have an overactive (hypertonic) pelvic floor, which needs the opposite approach. Do not start this protocol, see a pelvic floor physiotherapist first.

Commander's Briefing: Chapter 3

- **Three Tactics, One Engine:** The Synchronization Engine runs on The Reset (pelvic pre-fatigue), The Breath (coherence breathing), and The Rhythm (wave synchronization). Together, they give you complete control.

- **Tactic 1: The Reset is Non-Negotiable:** This is your foundation. Contract your pelvic floor maximally for 15-20 seconds before penetration. The muscle fatigue suppresses the ejaculatory reflex. Use mid-session Resets (12-15 second holds) when arousal builds.

- **Tactic 2: The Breath Maintains Calm:** Inhale for a slow count of five, exhale for a slow count of five. This coherence pattern keeps your nervous system in parasympathetic mode during penetration.

- **Tactic 3: The Rhythm Creates Art:** Nine shallow strokes, one deep. Or three shallow, one deep. The exact ratio matters less than the principle: predominantly shallow, occasionally deep. Avoid tensing during deep strokes.

- **The Hierarchy:** Tactic 1 alone provides significant control. Adding Tactic 2 amplifies control. Adding Tactic 3 achieves mastery. Build progressively; do not attempt all three simultaneously on first use.

- **The Mental Amplifier:** Believe you can hold. Think "I am in control, I choose when we finish." This mindset allows the technique to function optimally and builds the confidence that transforms your intimate life.

- **Individual Calibration Required:** Hold times, shallow/deep ratios, and Reset frequency will vary based on your physiology. Experiment during solo and partnered sessions to find your optimal parameters.

- **Erection and Ejaculation Are Separate Systems:** Your erection is maintained by blood flow (hydraulic). Ejaculation is triggered by muscle contraction (mechanical). Fatiguing your pelvic floor does not affect your erection. You remain fully aroused; only the reflex is disabled.

- **The Fatigue Window:** After a maximum contraction hold, your pelvic floor can only generate a fraction of its normal force. This is below the threshold required to trigger the ejaculatory reflex. Enter within 30 seconds of releasing your contraction to maximize this window.

- **Progressive Training Transforms Results:** A stronger pelvic floor means longer control windows between Resets. Beginners may need 3-5 Resets per session. Advanced practitioners often need only the initial pre-penetration Reset. Train consistently using the eight-week protocol in Appendix E: Pelvic Floor Training Fundamentals.

CHAPTER 4

THE PARTNER'S PLAYBOOK: FROM SOLO MISSION TO TEAM OPERATION

Three Conversations That Changed Everything

John's Sunday Morning

JOHN HAD REHEARSED THE words a hundred times. In the shower. On his commute. Lying awake at 2 AM while his girlfriend slept beside him.

I knew something was happening because I could see it from my kitchen window. John, my neighbor of three years, had started jogging at 6 AM. The software engineer who once joked that his only exercise was walking to the coffee machine was now running past my house every morning, rain or shine.

When I asked him about it over the fence one Saturday, he grinned. "The techniques are working," he said. "But my body couldn't keep up. I'm fixing that."

"And the conversation?" I asked. "Did you talk to her?"

His grin faded into something more vulnerable. "That's the hard part."

He chose a Sunday morning. They were on the couch, coffee in hand, nowhere to be. She was scrolling her phone, relaxed, unguarded.

"Hey," he said, his heart pounding harder than it had in any code review or product launch. "Can I talk to you about something?"

She looked up, a flicker of concern crossing her face. "Is everything okay?"

"Yeah. More than okay, actually." He set down his coffee. Took a breath. "I've been thinking a lot about us. About our intimacy. And I've been learning some techniques I'm really excited about."

Her eyebrows rose. This was not a conversation they had ever had.

"It's this system," he continued, "for being more present, more connected during... you know. For extending pleasure for both of us. Not tricks or anything weird. Just techniques for being better together."

She was quiet for a moment. Then: "You've been working on this?"

"A lot. And the thing is, it works best as a team. There's a whole approach designed for partners. About being a co-pilot."

"Co-pilot?" A small smile. "That sounds very... you."

"It is very me," he admitted. "But I want it to be very us."

She reached over and squeezed his hand. "Okay, engineer. Show me what you've got."

The conversation lasted an hour.

They talked about things they had never talked about. Fears. Desires.

The silence that had grown between them and why.

By the end, she was crying, and so was he.

"Why didn't we do this sooner?" she asked.

"I was scared," he said. "I thought you'd think I was broken."

She shook her head. "I think you're brave. And I think I'm really lucky."

That night, they practiced the *Breath Synchronization Drill*. No sex. Just breathing together, eyes locked, nervous systems slowly aligning. It was the most intimate experience of their relationship so far.

John texted me the next morning: "Why didn't anyone tell me talking was the unlock?"

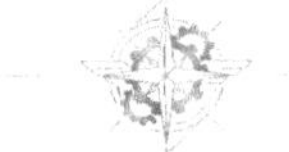

Matt's Surgical Approach

Matt approached the conversation the same way he approached everything: with meticulous preparation.

I had known Matt for two years through our kids' school. Our sons were in the same class, and we had spent countless hours on the sidelines of soccer games, making small talk about work and weather and the chaos of raising children. He was a trauma surgeon, brilliant and composed, the kind of man who seemed to have everything figured out.

Then came the parking lot conversation.

We were waiting for our kids after a school play. The other parents had drifted away. Matt stared at his phone, not really seeing it.

"Can I ask you something personal?" he said suddenly.

"Of course."

"How do you... talk to your wife about things that are hard to talk about?"

I knew immediately what he meant. Not because he said it, but because of the way he didn't.

I told him about the system. About what I had learned. About the conversation I'd had with my own wife. He listened without interrupting, the same focused attention he probably gave to surgical briefings.

"There's a chapter about this," I said. "About how to have the conversation. Would you want to read it?"

He nodded slowly. "I think I need to."

Two weeks later, Matt chose his moment. Friday evening, his son at a sleepover, a quiet dinner at home. He had planned the timing, the setting, even the words.

But when the moment came, the words evaporated.

His wife noticed. "What's wrong? You've been staring at your wine for ten minutes."

"Nothing's wrong." He paused. "Actually, I need to tell you something."

She set down her fork. Her face shifted into that careful neutrality he recognized from a thousand difficult conversations. "Okay."

"I've been learning something," he said. "About intimacy. About being more present. About…" He forced the words out. "About control. My control."

"Your control?"

"In bed. I've been struggling. For a while. And I've been hiding it because…" He looked at the table. "Because I didn't know how to talk about it. I command a trauma unit, for God's sake. I hold hearts in my hands. And I can't…"

He could not finish the sentence.

The silence stretched. When he finally looked up, his wife's eyes were wet.

"Matt," she said quietly. "I know."

"You know?"

"Of course I know. I've known for years." She reached across the table. "I just didn't know how to bring it up without hurting you. You carry so much. I didn't want to add to it."

Something broke open in Matt's chest. All the shame he had carried, the isolation, the feeling that he was fighting alone, she had been on the other side of that wall the whole time, waiting for him to knock.

"I'm sorry," he said. "I should have talked to you."

"We're talking now." She squeezed his hand. "Tell me everything."

He told her. About *The Reset*. About the breathing. About the partner's role. She listened without interrupting, her grip on his hand never loosening.

"So I'm supposed to be a co-pilot?" she asked when he finished.

"If you want to be."

"Matt." She smiled for the first time in what felt like months. "I've been waiting in the cockpit for years. I was starting to think you'd never let me help fly."

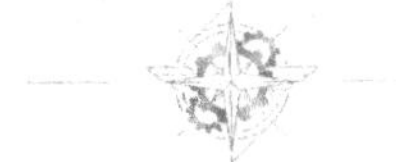

David's Organic Unfolding

David did not plan the conversation. It happened the way most important things happen in a fifteen-year marriage: organically, unexpectedly, in the small hours when defenses are down.

David was my oldest friend, someone I had known since before either of us had mortgages or children or the particular exhaustion that comes with both. We had watched each other's lives unfold, celebrated the victories, supported each other through the setbacks.

So when he called me one afternoon, his voice strange, I knew something had shifted.

"She made a joke," he said without preamble.

"Who? About what?"

"My wife. Last night. After we..." He trailed off. "She said, 'For that, I probably didn't need to take off my pants.'"

I waited.

"She laughed after she said it. Like it was just a joke. But I've been thinking about it all day." His voice cracked slightly. "She's been telling me something for years, hasn't she? And I've been too stupid to hear it."

I told him about the system. Sent him the materials. Encouraged him to read the chapter about the conversation.

"I don't think I need to plan some big talk," he said. "I think it's going to happen on its own."

He was right.

A few nights later, they were lying in bed. The lights were off, but neither of them was sleeping. The joke hung in the air between them, unaddressed but present.

"I want to talk about what you said," David started.

She turned to face him. "What I said?"

"The pants thing."

She winced. "David, I was kidding. I didn't mean…"

"No." He held up a hand. "You meant it. And you were right to say it."

She was quiet.

"I've been thinking about it constantly," he continued. "About how long I've been… not enough. In this area. And I always told myself it was normal. That every guy was like me. But that's not true, is it?"

"David…"

"I found something. A method. A real system for this." He turned to look at her directly. "And I want to try it. But it works best with a partner. As a team."

She studied his face in the dim light. "You've been researching this?"

"Seriously researching. There are exercises for couples. Drills. Ways to communicate without words. Ways to…"

"Ways to make me not need to joke about keeping my pants on?"

Despite the tension, he laughed. She always could do that, defuse things with humor. It was her gift, and sometimes her weapon.

"Yeah. Exactly that."

She propped herself up on one elbow. A slow smile spread across her face. "After fifteen years, we're going to practice?"

"I want to learn to be what you deserve," he said. "And I can't do it alone."

She leaned over and kissed him. Soft. Unhurried. The first kiss in months that felt like it meant something.

"Let's start tonight," she said. "Show me one of these exercises."

They tried the *Sensory Mapping Drill*. David, the man who commanded construction sites, spent twenty minutes tracing his fingertip across his wife's shoulders, her back, the curve of her hip, listening for each whispered "yes."

When they finished, she looked at him differently. Like she was seeing someone she had forgotten was there.

"Fifteen years," she said. "And you can still surprise me."

David texted me the next day: "I think we just started over. In a good way."

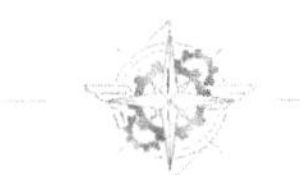

The Most Difficult Conversation

For a man who can negotiate a multi-million dollar contract without flinching, who can lead a team through a crisis with a steady hand, one of the most terrifying prospects can be a single, quiet conversation with the person who matters most.

You have trained your mind like a commander and calibrated your body like a high-performance machine. The keys to the *Synchronization Engine* are now in your hands. But even the most skilled pilot reaches peak potential when a talented *Co-Pilot* navigates by their side, reading the map, watching for blind spots, and managing the systems so the pilot can focus on flying. Flying solo is possible. Flying as a team is where true mastery is found.

This chapter is about transforming this journey from a "me" task into a "we" mission.

The *Tactical Intimacy System* is not a "problem" for a man to solve in secret shame. It is a skill upgrade for a couple to explore together, a new language of pleasure and connection. Your partner is your greatest ally in this process: your most honest source of real-time feedback and the biggest celebrator of your success. Enlisting her in this mission will not just double the results; it will multiply them.

This conversation is the gateway.

However, this is a delicate operation. Approached incorrectly, it can be disastrous. Approached correctly, with the tactical precision of a commander, it can elevate your relationship to a level of honesty, playfulness, and passion you have never experienced before.

The Man's Briefing: How to Initiate the Conversation

Setting the Commander's Intent for Communication

Before you say a single word, you must be crystal clear on your intent. This is not a confession. This is not an apology. Opening up to your partner about this is not an admission of weakness. It is a demonstration of profound strength, a testament to how much you value her pleasure, and a declaration that you are willing to invest in making your shared intimacy extraordinary.

You are not presenting a problem. You are presenting an opportunity. You are inviting her to join you in building something remarkable.

True command is not about having no weaknesses. It is about having the courage to address them strategically.

Relationship researcher Dr. John Gottman has studied couples for over four decades in his "Love Lab" at the University of Washington. His research revealed something remarkable: he can predict with remarkable accuracy whether a couple will stay together or separate, based largely on how a difficult conversation begins. The single biggest factor? Whether the conversation begins with a *Harsh Start-Up*, blame, criticism, "You always...," or what he calls a *Soft Start-Up*, taking responsibility, expressing a need, using "I feel..." statements.

Your approach here is a Soft Start-Up for the most important project of all: your relationship.

The Invitation Approach vs. The Harsh Start-up

The Wrong Approach (Harsh Start-up):

"Hey, we need to talk. I have a problem with premature ejaculation, and I am reading a book to fix it."

This immediately frames the topic as a negative "problem" that you have been hiding. It uses "I," which isolates you and makes it sound like your secret burden. It can instantly make your partner feel insecure, implicated, or defensive. The conversation starts in a hole you will have to dig yourself out of.

The Right Approach (*The Invitation Approach*):

"Hey, can we chat for a minute? I have been thinking a lot about our intimacy and how amazing it is, and I have come across some incredible ideas for how we can make it even more fun and passionate. It is all about new techniques focused on extending pleasure and connection for both of us, and honestly, I would be really excited to explore them with you. I would love for you to be my co-pilot on this adventure."

This starts with a positive affirmation. It uses "we" and "us," making it a team mission from the first sentence. It frames the topic as an exciting "adventure" and an "exploration," not a problem to be solved. And it explicitly invites her to be your "co-pilot," giving her a powerful, respected, and integral role. You are not asking for help. You are inviting her to join the flight crew.

Rules of Engagement

Timing and Terrain. Do not have this conversation right after a frustrating sexual encounter, late at night when you are both tired, or in the middle of a stressful week. Those are moments when defenses are high and emotional reserves are low. Choose a neutral, relaxed time. A walk after dinner. A quiet moment on a weekend morning with coffee. Relaxing on the couch together, free of deadlines and distractions. The environment dictates the mood.

Focus on the "Why." Your "why" is not "so I can last longer." That is a mechanical outcome. Your "why" is the emotional and relational benefit. Use phrases like: "so we can connect more deeply," "so I can focus entirely on your pleasure without being in my head," "so we can unlock new levels of passion together." Always frame the benefit in terms of the partnership.

Invite, Do Not Instruct. You are not giving her a new set of instructions or a performance review. The energy should be collaborative, not managerial. You are inviting her to join a mission. Use language like: "Would you be open to trying something new with me?" or "I would love your help with this. It sounds like it could be really fun." or "What do you think about us exploring this together?"

Show, Do Not Just Tell. If she is receptive, you can say: "This book I am reading has a whole chapter written specifically for you, as the co-pilot. It actually frames the partner as the most important part of the whole system. Would you be interested in reading it?" This shows that she is a central, respected part of the system, not an afterthought.

Be Prepared to Listen. This is not a monologue. After you extend the invitation, stop talking. Let her react. She might have questions, concerns, or feel a mix of emotions. Your job now is to practice the TIS principle of calm presence. Listen to understand, not to rebut. This conversation is the first test of your new skills outside the bedroom.

When the Conversation Does Not Go as Planned

Not every partner will immediately embrace this journey with you. This is normal and does not mean the relationship is doomed or that you cannot make progress.

If Your Partner is Hesitant: Hesitation is not rejection. She may need time to process. She may have her own insecurities about intimacy that your invitation has surfaced. She may simply be surprised. Respect her pace completely. Do not pressure or create ultimatums. Say: "I understand. There is no rush. I just wanted you to know what I am working on, and the door is always open." Focus on the solo training aspects: breathing, The Reset, mindset. Lead by example. Let her see the positive changes in your overall demeanor, your presence, your patience. Revisit the conversation later, with patience, when the moment feels right.

If Your Partner is Resistant or Dismissive: This is more challenging, but not insurmountable. Consider whether there are underlying relationship issues that need attention first. Intimacy problems are often symptoms, not causes. A couples therapist can provide a safe, neutral space to discuss sensitive topics. This is not failure; it is wisdom. Remember: you cannot control her response. You can only control your own growth. Continue your solo practice. The improvements in your presence, confidence, and patience will speak louder than any conversation.

Important: If attempts to discuss intimacy consistently result in conflict or emotional distress for either partner, this may indicate deeper issues that benefit from professional guidance. There is no shame in seeking help. The strongest couples are often those who have done the work with a skilled guide.

The Partner's Playbook: The Co-Pilot's Role

(This section is written to be shared. The highest-level TIS operators encourage their partners to read this.)

Welcome, Co-pilot.

The man in your life has just paid you the highest compliment: he has invited you into the engine room of his inner world. He has chosen to be vulnerable, to share a goal, and to declare that this mission of creating extraordinary intimacy is one he cannot, and does not want to, complete without you.

It is a sign of his profound commitment to you and his trust in your partnership.

His journey to master the Tactical Intimacy System is a testament to how deeply he cares about you and your shared pleasure. Your role in this process is not just supportive; it is vital. You are the mission's lead navigator, the primary source of intelligence, and the key to unlocking the full potential of your teamwork.

He can learn to fly the plane. But you are the one who knows the destination.

Your Role: The Navigator

A pilot without a navigator flies blind. He can keep the aircraft in the air, but he cannot see the weather ahead, the terrain below, or the optimal route to the destination. You are the one who knows the terrain. You read the conditions he cannot read from the cockpit. Your voice, your signals, your feedback are what transform a solo flight into a shared journey.

This is not a passive role. A navigator makes critical decisions in real time: when to adjust course, when to climb, when to descend, when to say "hold steady, this is perfect." Without your input, he is guessing. With it, he is flying with precision and confidence.

Your feedback is not a favor you do for him. It is the essential data that makes the entire system work. When you tell him what feels good, what you want more of, what to slow down or speed up, you are not just helping him. You are co-creating an experience that belongs to both of you.

Acknowledge the Invitation

The first and most important step is to recognize what just happened. For many men, initiating this conversation is one of the hardest things they will ever do. He chose to trust you with something most men carry in silence for years, sometimes decades.

A simple, heartfelt response is the most powerful fuel you can give him: "Thank you for sharing this with me. It means a lot that you trust me with this. I am excited and honored to do this together."

These words cost nothing and give everything.

Provide Experiential, Not Performance-Based, Feedback

He is rewiring his brain to move away from performance anxiety. Your feedback is critical to this process. The stopwatch is the enemy.

Performance Feedback (Less Helpful): "You lasted longer that time." This still keeps the focus on time and performance metrics. It reinforces the very anxiety he is trying to escape.

Experiential Feedback (Transformative): "That slow, deliberate rhythm you used was incredible. It made me feel so connected to you and so desired." Or: "When I could feel you breathing with me, it was a total turn-on." Or: "I love how focused you were on me just then. It made me feel like I was the only person in the world."

This kind of feedback rewards the process, not just the outcome. It reinforces the very behaviors he is trying to learn. And it will make both of you feel incredible.

Create a Pressure-Free Zone

Treat your practice sessions not as an exam, but as a playground for exploration. Be playful. Laugh if something feels awkward. Initiate sessions with the explicit goal of "just practicing," with no expectation of orgasm for either of you.

You can even create a fun code word for it. "Time for a training mission." "Let us go to the lab." "Research and development night."

Pressure is the primary enemy of the TIS. Your encouragement and light-heartedness are its greatest antidote.

Creating a Safe Training Ground: Drills for Two

Mastery requires practice. Together, you can turn this practice into a fun, intimate, and deeply bonding experience. These are not clinical exercises. They are opportunities to rediscover each other, to communicate without words, and to build anticipation for what comes next.

The Sensory Mapping Drill

This drill shifts his focus from performance to sensory intelligence, and opens new pathways of pleasure for both of you.

The Setup: Choose a time when you will not be interrupted. Dim the lights. Put on music that relaxes you both. One of you is the "Mapper" (the one giving touch), the other is the "Navigator" (the one receiving). The Navigator lies down in a comfortable, warm space. Clothing is optional, but less is more for this exercise. The vulnerability is part of the experience.

The Mission: The Mapper's goal is to use a single fingertip to slowly and lightly trace lines across the Navigator's body: back, arms, legs, neck, the curve of the hip, the inside of the wrist. Move slowly. There is nowhere to be. The Navigator's job is to close their eyes and simply say "yes" whenever a touch feels particularly good or interesting. No other words. No explanations. Just a simple, soft "yes."

For the Mapper: Pay attention. Where does "yes" come? How does her breathing change in certain areas? Notice the slight arch of her back, the way her skin responds to different pressures. You are learning her map.

For the Navigator: Surrender to the sensation. Do not think about whether your "yes" is in the right place. Trust your body. Let yourself be discovered.

The Debrief: After ten to fifteen minutes, switch roles. When you have both been Mapper and Navigator, talk about what you discovered. What surprised you? What did you learn about each other? This exercise trains him to focus on external feedback. It trains you both in the art of non-verbal communication. And it often leads to places neither of you expected.

The Breath Synchronization Drill

This connects directly to the core of the TIS Method and builds a profound sense of physiological and emotional connection.

The Setup: Sit facing each other, cross-legged on the floor or on a bed, close enough so your knees are almost touching. You can place your hands on each other's shoulders, hold hands, or simply rest them on your own knees with eyes connected. The lighting should be soft. Eye contact is essential.

The Mission: One of you starts the *Coherence Breathing* pattern: inhale through your nose for a slow count of five, exhale through your nose for a slow count of five. The other's mission is to synchronize. Feel his chest rise as yours does. Fall as his falls. Watch his eyes. Notice how his shoulders drop as he exhales. Match him. Become him. After a minute, let the roles blur. You are no longer leading or following. You are simply breathing together. Continue for five minutes. Do not speak.

The Goal: The aim is to feel your nervous systems calming down together. This is a powerful, non-verbal way of saying: "We are a team. We are in sync." This drill is the perfect warm-up for a practice session. It calms both of you, unites your focus, and creates a sense of intimacy before a single piece of clothing comes off. Many couples report that this exercise alone transforms their connection.

Establish Non-Verbal Cues

In the heat of the moment, words can feel disruptive. They can pull you out of the experience and back into your head. Agree on a set of simple, non-verbal signals you can use during intimacy.

Make it a fun, collaborative project to decide on these together. Here are some examples to start: a gentle squeeze of his hand for "a little slower." A specific light scratch on his shoulder for "do not stop, that is perfect." A double tap on his hip for "I am close." Pulling him deeper for "more." A soft push on his chest for "pause, I need a moment."

These signals allow you to communicate and guide the experience without breaking the spell. They keep you both present, connected, and responsive to each other's needs in real time.

> ## The Journey Beyond Technique
>
> This process will do more than increase control and pleasure in the bedroom. It will strengthen the muscles of communication, trust, and teamwork that are the foundation of a resilient relationship.
>
> You will learn to talk about things that once felt impossible to discuss. You will discover new dimensions of each other. You will build a private language that belongs only to the two of you.
>
> The couples who master the TIS Method often report that the benefits extend far beyond intimacy. They communicate better about everything. They feel more connected in daily life. They laugh more. They fight less. This is the hidden gift of the work you are doing together.
>
> For couple exercises, conversation starters, and planning templates, see Appendix F: The Connection Toolkit. For digital tools designed to support your practice as a couple, visit tismethod.com/tactical-intimacy/book-owners .

Commander's Q&A: Navigating the Conversation

What if I bring this up and she gets defensive or insecure?

This is a possibility, often rooted in her own fears: *Am I not enough?* If this happens, do not get defensive in return. Your mission is to reassure. Your mantra should be: "This has absolutely nothing to do with you being anything less than amazing. This is about me wanting to be a better, more present partner for you. My goal is to give you even more pleasure and for us to have more fun together." Reiterate that it is a team project, an upgrade for the partnership, not a bug fix for you.

My partner and I do not really talk about sex in this way. It feels awkward.

The initial awkwardness is the barrier to entry for a new level of intimacy. Acknowledge it directly. You can say: "I know we do not usually talk this openly, and it feels a bit uncomfortable to even bring this up. But I think what is on the other side of this conversation is so worth it for us." Naming the awkwardness instantly reduces its power. It shows you are both in it together. It is like the first day at a new gym: uncomfortable until it becomes familiar.

Will focusing so much on technique kill the passion?

Only if you remain stuck in the "learning" phase forever. Think of a seasoned pilot. He has spent thousands of hours in simulators and training flights, mastering instruments, emergency procedures, and navigation systems. But when he is in the air, he is not reciting checklists. He is reading the sky, feeling the aircraft, responding to conditions with fluid confidence. The hours of technical mastery have become invisible, freeing him to fly with instinct and grace. The TIS Method works the same way. The practice you do together is like learning the instruments. Eventually, the instruments disappear into the flight. And the flight becomes more beautiful than either of you imagined.

Commander's Briefing: Chapter 4

- **Mission Objective: Upgrade from Solo to Team.** This is not your problem to solve in secret. Transform this journey from a "me" task into a "we" mission. Your partner is your greatest ally; enlist her as your co-pilot.

- **Initiating the Conversation is a Tactical Operation.** Your approach determines the outcome. The Harsh Start-up, "I have a problem and I am fixing it," creates blame, insecurity, and defensiveness. The Invitation Approach, "I have been learning how we can make our intimacy even more incredible, and I want you to be my co-pilot on this adventure," frames it as an exciting, shared upgrade.

- **Rules of Engagement for the Talk:** Timing is everything; choose a neutral, relaxed moment. Frame the benefit for "us," not "me." Invite, do not instruct. Collaborative language only.

- **The Co-pilot's Playbook (Your Partner's Role):** She is your navigator, not a passive supporter. Her feedback is the essential data that makes the system work. Experiential feedback ("that rhythm made me feel incredible") rewires his brain faster than performance metrics ("you lasted longer"). A pressure-free zone turns practice into play.

- **Three Proven Approaches Exist:** Planned (structured timing and setting), responsive (seizing an organic moment of vulnerability), and spontaneous (letting the conversation emerge naturally). All three work when framed as an invitation, not a confession.

- **Your Partner May Already Know.** Do not assume you are hiding anything. Assume she has been hoping you would trust her enough to share.

- **Shared Training Drills:** The Sensory Mapping Drill teaches focused touch and non-verbal communication. The Breath Synchronization Drill physically and emotionally syncs your nervous systems before intimacy begins. Non-Verbal Cues create a silent language to guide each other without breaking presence.

- **If She Is Not Ready:** Respect her pace. Continue your solo practice. Lead by example. Revisit later with patience. If resistance persists, consider professional guidance. The strongest couples are often those who have done the work with a skilled guide.

CHAPTER 5

THE ENDURANCE TACTIC: BUILDING THE HIGH-PERFORMANCE CHASSIS

Why Your Body Matters

YOU MAY BE WONDERING: *I bought a book about sexual performance. Why am I reading about cardiovascular fitness and squats?*

The greatest breathing technique in the world cannot compensate for a body that runs out of steam after five minutes.

Sexual intercourse is, at its core, a physical activity. It requires cardiovascular endurance to maintain rhythm without gasping for breath. It requires muscular strength in your hips, core, and legs to sustain movement and explore different positions. It requires flexibility to access positions that maximize pleasure for both partners.

A man who masters the TIS breathing techniques but neglects his physical conditioning is like a Formula 1 driver with perfect technique in a car with a weak engine. The skills are there, but the chassis cannot deliver.

Moreover, physical fitness directly impacts your hormonal environment. Regular exercise naturally optimizes testosterone levels, reduces the cortisol that kills desire, and floods your system with endorphins that enhance mood and confidence.

In the previous chapters, we built the high-performance engine of the *Tactical Intimacy System*. You have synchronized your mind, breath, and muscles to achieve an unprecedented level of control. You have enlisted your partner as a co-pilot for your shared mission. The software is installed and running flawlessly.

Now it is time to build the chassis that will carry that engine, allow it to unleash its full power, and keep you in the race for the long haul. This is not about vanity or ego. This is about capability and command.

Three Men, Three Journeys

John's Awakening

John had started jogging at 6 AM, a transformation I described in the previous chapter. What I did not mention was why.

The first time he implemented the TIS techniques with his girlfriend, he felt the difference immediately. The mental clarity was there. The control was working. But ten minutes into physical intimacy, something else became impossible to ignore.

He was gasping like he had just sprinted up ten flights of stairs.

His arms trembled when he held himself above her. His lower back screamed in protest. Sweat poured down his face, not from passion, but from exertion. And the next morning, his body ached in places he did not know could ache.

"You okay?" his girlfriend had asked, watching him wince as he reached for his coffee.

"Just slept weird," he lied.

The truth was harder to admit: his body had betrayed him. At 28, he should have been in his prime. Instead, years of desk work and takeout dinners had left him physically unprepared for the demands of extended intimacy.

John started small, the way engineers approach any problem. A 20-minute jog three times a week. Basic bodyweight exercises in his living room while his code compiled. Push-ups. Squats. Planks that made him shake and curse.

The first two weeks were brutal. His legs burned. His lungs protested. He questioned whether this was worth it.

Then, around week three, something shifted.

The jogs became easier. The push-ups stopped feeling like torture. And in the bedroom, the change was unmistakable.

He could hold himself above her without his arms trembling. He could maintain rhythm without gasping for air. He could be present, fully present, because his body was no longer screaming for attention.

But the most surprising change was something he had not expected at all.

His erections were different. Harder. Faster to arrive. Longer to fade. The combination of cardiovascular fitness and the TIS techniques created a synergy he had not anticipated.

His girlfriend noticed too.

"Whatever you're doing," she said one night, lying beside him in the afterglow, "keep doing it."

John texted me the next morning: "Why didn't anyone tell me the gym was foreplay?"

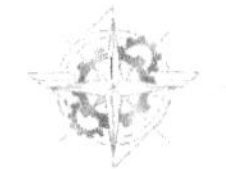

Matt's Reckoning

Matt's transformation started with a number he did not want to hear.

We were at a school event for our kids, our sons were in the same class, when he mentioned, almost casually, that his doctor had flagged his visceral fat levels during a routine physical. "He said something I can't stop thinking about," Matt told me, keeping his voice low so other parents would not overhear. "That the belly fat isn't just sitting there. It's metabolically active. Converting testosterone to estrogen."

I watched his face as he processed what that meant. Here was a man who held beating hearts in his hands, who made split-second decisions in the operating room, learning that his own body had been sabotaging him for years. "I blamed age," he said. "I blamed stress. I blamed the impossible hours. But the real problem was sitting right around my waist the entire time."

Matt had a different challenge than John. He was on his feet for twelve-hour shifts. He walked miles through hospital corridors. He assumed that counted as exercise.

It did not.

Years of hospital cafeteria food, stress eating during overnight calls, and no time for the gym had taken their toll. The extra twenty pounds around his midsection were not just cosmetic. They were actively working against him, converting the very hormone he needed into one he did not.

He committed to two strength sessions per week. Nothing heroic. Thirty minutes in the hospital gym before his shift, while the building was still quiet. Squats. Deadlifts. Planks. The movements felt awkward at first, his surgeon's hands more accustomed to delicate instruments than barbells.

He cleaned up his diet. Meal prep on Sundays. Protein and vegetables instead of whatever the cafeteria was serving. He stopped stress-eating during overnight calls, replacing the vending machine runs with walks around the hospital perimeter.

The first month, he lost eight pounds. The second month, another seven. But the numbers on the scale were not the real victory. The real victory was what he felt. Energy he had not experienced in years. Desire that arrived unbidden, surprising him in the middle of ordinary moments. Morning erections that had become rare visitors were now reliable guests.

His wife noticed before he said anything.

"You seem... different," she said one evening, watching him move around the kitchen with an energy she had not seen in years.

"Different how?"

"Lighter. More... here."

She was right. He was more present. More alive. The fog that had settled over his life was lifting, and underneath it, he found a version of himself he had forgotten existed.

At a school pickup a few weeks later, Matt pulled me aside.

"What I thought was 'getting older,'" he said, "turned out to be a body fighting against itself. Once I stopped the fight, everything changed."

David's Physical Plateau

David called me one afternoon, frustrated in a way I had rarely heard from him.

"My back gave out," he said. "Last night.

With my wife. We were trying something we've done a hundred times, and my body just... quit."

David had been fit enough for years. Weekend warrior basketball games. Occasional gym visits.

At 41, he could still keep up, mostly.

But he noticed things changing. Recovery took longer. The morning after basketball, his knees ached in ways they never had at thirty.

And in the bedroom, positions that once felt natural now left him winded or caused his lower back to seize.

The wake-up call came during that intimate moment with his wife. They were trying a position they had enjoyed for years when his lower back locked up.

Not dramatically, not painfully, but enough that he had to stop, roll onto his back, and spend the next minute stretching while his wife looked on with concern and barely concealed frustration.

"Getting old," he joked. But the joke felt hollow.

His wife said nothing. She did not have to. The moment was over. The connection broken. Another evening that ended in disappointment rather than connection.

David started small. Not a gym membership he would abandon in three weeks, but simple mobility work at home. Hip openers he found on YouTube. Core exercises he could do in his living room. Stretches that targeted the lower back that had betrayed him.

The first month felt pointless. He was not losing weight or building visible muscle. But he kept going. By month two, something shifted. The basketball games got easier. His knees stopped screaming the next morning. He moved differently, more fluidly, more confidently.

And in the bedroom?

The change was profound. He could hold positions without thinking about his back. He could transition smoothly without stopping to stretch. He could focus entirely on his wife because his body was no longer a distraction.

"I forgot what my body was capable of," he told his wife one evening after a particularly satisfying encounter. "I just needed to remind it."

She smiled. "Welcome back."

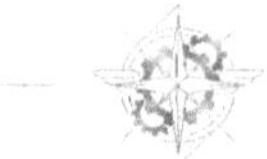

The Kingdom of Cardio: The Heart of Sexual Performance

Blood Flow is Everything

At its most fundamental, physiological level, sexual performance rests on one undeniable reality: blood flow. A strong, healthy erection is nothing more and nothing less than a hydraulic event, made possible by blood rushing into and being trapped within the penis. Sustained sexual intercourse is an athletic event that depends on your heart's ability to efficiently pump oxygenated blood throughout your body.

Your cardiovascular health is not an abstract concept for a doctor's office; it is the absolute foundation of your sexual power. Every minute you spend on the treadmill, on the bike, or in the pool is not just about burning calories; it is a direct training session for the bedroom.

It Boosts Stamina and Eliminates the Breathlessness Barrier. Regular cardio strengthens your heart muscle and increases your lung capacity (your *VO2 max*). You tire less quickly during physical exertion. Think about a moment when you were physically intimate and suddenly became aware of your own ragged breathing. In that instant, your focus shifted from your partner to your own fatigue. You were pulled out of the moment and into your head. When your body is efficient, your mind can remain calm and in command, fully present with your partner.

It Clears the Pipes for Harder Erections. Aerobic exercise is the single best thing you can do for your vascular system. It helps keep your blood vessels flexible, elastic, and clear of the plaque that can stiffen and narrow them over time. Think of your circulatory system as a network of highways. A sedentary lifestyle creates traffic jams and roadblocks: plaque buildup and endothelial dysfunction. Cardio is the road crew that works around the clock, keeping those highways wide open and free of debris, ensuring blood can rush to where it is needed most, exactly when it is needed. This process is heavily reliant on the production of *Nitric Oxide* (*NO*), a gas molecule that acts as the master signal for your blood vessels to relax and widen. Cardio exercise is a potent stimulator of NO production, making it a natural and powerful erection booster.

It Is a Natural Antidote to Stress. The stress hormone cortisol triggers your Fight or Flight response and is a passion killer. Cardio is nature's most powerful stress reducer. It burns off excess cortisol and releases a cascade of endorphins, your brain's natural *feel-good* chemicals. A man who regularly exercises is calmer, more confident, and less prone to the anxiety that sabotages performance. He enters the bedroom with a clean slate, not carrying the physical and mental weight of his day.

Your Weekly Cardio Mission

The goal here is consistency, not heroism. You do not need to train for a marathon.

Sample Weekly Plan:

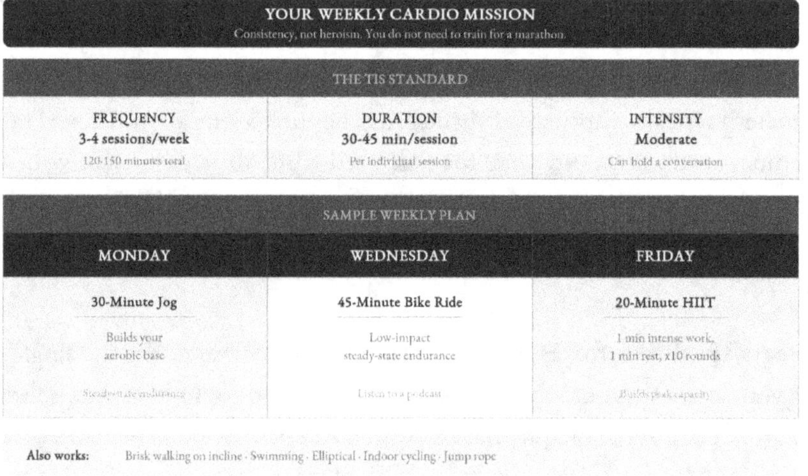

Functional Strength: Training for the Real World

Performance Muscles vs. Beach Muscles

The goal of TIS strength training is not to look like you belong on the cover of a bodybuilding magazine (though that may be a pleasant side effect). The goal is to perform the specific, functional movements of intercourse with more power, more control, more variety, and less risk of injury.

Many men focus on *beach muscles*, biceps, chest, and abs. While aesthetically pleasing, these are not the muscles that drive sexual performance. A sports car with a huge, powerful engine is useless if its transmission and drivetrain are weak. We need to train the drivetrain.

Hips and Lower Back (Glutes and Core): Your Power Plant

These are your thrusting engines. The power for deep, rhythmic, and controlled movement does not come from your arms or your chest; it originates in your hips and is stabilized by your core. Strong glutes and a stable lower back allow for movements that are not only more powerful but also more fluid and less taxing on your body. Weakness here leads to fatigue, poor form, and potential injury. Key exercises: Barbell Squats, Deadlifts, Kettlebell Swings, and Hip Thrusts are the undisputed kings for building raw power in this region. They also trigger a significant release of testosterone and growth hormone, further enhancing your vitality.

The Core: Your Center of Stability

Your core (the complex of muscles around your midsection, including your abs, obliques, and lower back) is your body's center of balance and force transfer. A strong core provides stability in a wide variety of sexual positions, dramatically reduces the load and potential for strain on your lower back, and allows for smooth, controlled transitions between movements. It is the solid platform upon which all movement is built. Without a strong core, the power from your hips is wasted. Key exercises: Planks (and their variations), Leg Raises, and Russian Twists are perfect for building a core of solid, functional steel.

Flexibility: The Key to Freedom

Flexibility is the most overlooked and undervalued component of male fitness. It is the key to variety, comfort, and injury prevention. A flexible body has a greater range of motion, allowing you and your partner to comfortably explore a wider array of positions without strain. If you have ever thought, *I cannot hold that position for long*, it is often a flexibility issue, not a strength one. Flexibility unlocks new pages in your intimate playbook. Key practices: Simple static stretching after each workout, or a dedicated 15-20 minute weekly yoga or mobility session, can create a revolution in your physical freedom.

Training for Specific Scenarios

Without naming specific positions, here is how different muscle groups translate to bedroom capability.

TRAINING FOR SPECIFIC SCENARIOS

How Your Gym Work Translates to the Bedroom

SCENARIO	PRIMARY MUSCLES	KEY EXERCISES
Supporting your weight above your partner	Chest, shoulders, triceps, core	Push-ups, Bench Press, Plank
Kneeling and thrusting power and rhythm	Quadriceps, glutes, hip flexors	Squats, Lunges, Hip Thrusts
Standing and supporting your partner's weight	Full legs, core, grip strength	Deadlifts, Farmer's Walks
Side-lying sustained movement and control	Hip abductors, obliques	Side Plank, Clamshells
Flexibility for variety range of motion	Hamstrings, hip flexors, lower back	Butterfly, Pigeon Pose, Deep Squat

Your Weekly Mission: 2-3 full-body strength sessions per week
The more physically capable you are, the more options you have.

The more physically capable you are, the more options you have. The more options you have, the more varied and exciting your intimate life becomes.

Your Weekly Strength Mission

Aim for 2-3 full-body strength sessions per week, focusing on compound movements that mimic real-world actions.

Sample TIS Strength Workout:

SAMPLE TIS STRENGTH WORKOUT		
2-3 full-body sessions per week · Compound movements · Functional power		
EXERCISE	SETS x REPS	WHY IT MATTERS
Barbell Squats or Goblet Squats	3 x 8-10	Ultimate leg and glute builder for powerful hip drive
Push-ups or Bench Press	3 x 8-10	Upper body strength for weight-bearing positions
Deadlifts or KB Swings	3 x 10-12	Posterior chain power and explosive strength
Plank	3 x max hold	Core stability and lower back health
Post-Workout Stretching	10 min	Hamstrings, hips (pigeon pose), lower back

Focus on compound movements. Train the drivetrain, not just the armor.
These exercises also trigger testosterone and growth hormone release, enhancing your vitality.

The Fuel Tank: Nutrition for Performance

You can have the best car in the world, with the most powerful engine and the strongest chassis, but if you put low-quality fuel in the tank, the engine will sputter and fail. Your body works the same way. What you eat directly affects your energy levels, your hormone production, your mood, and your circulatory health.

Tactical Nutrients

Support Testosterone. Testosterone is the primary hormone of the male libido and drive. A diet rich in zinc (found in red meat, shellfish, pumpkin seeds), Vitamin D (sunlight, fatty fish), and healthy fats (avocado, olive oil, nuts) helps keep your testosterone levels in their optimal range.

Increase Blood Flow (Nitric Oxide Boosters). Foods rich in nitrates, like leafy greens (spinach, arugula), beets, and pomegranate, are converted into Nitric Oxide (NO) in the body. NO is the crucial molecule that helps dilate your blood vessels, directly improving blood flow and erection quality. Watermelon, rich in L-citrulline, is another potent NO-booster. For four concentrated drink recipes designed to maximize these compounds, see Appendix B: TIS Performance Drinks.

Energy and Stamina. Complex carbohydrates like oats, sweet potatoes, and brown rice provide slow-release energy, fueling you for longer sessions without the crash that comes from sugar and refined carbs.

The Saboteurs: What to Eliminate

Processed Foods and Sugar

Highly processed foods, sugary drinks, and trans fats sap your energy, cause inflammation, and over time, damage the delicate lining of your blood vessels (the endothelium), impeding blood flow.

Visceral Fat: The Biochemistry You Need to Understand

That belly fat is not inert tissue. Visceral fat (the fat around your midsection and organs) produces an enzyme called *aromatase*. This enzyme converts your testosterone into estrogen. The more visceral fat you carry, the more testosterone your body converts to estrogen through this process. This is not a character flaw. It is biochemistry. And biochemistry can be changed.

This is why men with significant visceral fat often experience lower libido, weaker erections, and reduced energy. Reducing your waist circumference is one of the most powerful things you can do for your sexual health.

Smoking

Smoking is the number one destroyer of erections. Nicotine constricts your blood vessels immediately upon entering your system. Over time, the chemicals in cigarettes cause permanent damage to the delicate walls of your arteries, making them stiff and unable to dilate properly. The small arteries in the penis are among the first to be affected. Many men experiencing erectile dysfunction in their 30s and

40s can trace the problem directly back to their smoking history. If you smoke, quitting is the single most impactful thing you can do for your sexual health. Nothing else comes close.

Excessive Alcohol

While a single glass of wine can be a relaxant, excessive alcohol consumption is a triple threat: it lowers testosterone, depresses the central nervous system (making it harder to maintain arousal), and leads to dehydration, which reduces stamina and blood volume. The belief that alcohol improves performance is a myth. It only temporarily reduces inhibition while simultaneously sabotaging the physical mechanisms you need.

Oral Health

Men with gum disease (periodontitis) are significantly more likely to experience erectile dysfunction. The reason is systemic inflammation. The bacteria from infected gums enter your bloodstream and cause inflammation throughout your vascular system, including the small vessels in your penis. Daily flossing and regular dental care are not just about fresh breath. They are about protecting your entire circulatory system.

The Recovery Factor: Sleep as a Performance Enhancer

There is a fourth pillar that most men completely ignore: recovery. Specifically, sleep.

Your body produces the majority of its testosterone during deep sleep, particularly during REM cycles. This is not a minor detail. It is the primary manufacturing window for the hormone that drives your desire, your energy, and your erections.

Additionally, during sleep, you experience nocturnal erections. These are not random; they are your body's way of testing the system and oxygenating penile tissue. Men who consistently get poor sleep often notice weaker morning erections, a direct indicator of reduced overnight maintenance.

The TIS Sleep Standard:

THE TIS SLEEP STANDARD		
Sleep is not laziness. It is active recovery.		
DURATION	QUALITY	CONSISTENCY
7-9 hours	Dark room	Same sleep time
uninterrupted sleep per night	Cool temperature	Same wake time
	No screens 30 min before bed	Even on weekends
Testosterone is produced during deep REM cycles	Nocturnal erections oxygenate penile tissue during quality sleep	Irregular sleep disrupts hormonal production cycles

A man who sleeps well performs well. There are no shortcuts around this.
Poor sleep weakens morning erections, a direct indicator of reduced overnight maintenance.

See Chapter 6: Evening Wind-Down Protocol for your pre-sleep routine.

For performance drink recipes designed to support blood flow and hormonal health, see Appendix B: TIS Performance Drinks. For digital resources, visit tismethod.com/tactical-intimacy/book-owners.

Commander's Q&A: Overcoming Resistance

I do not have time to go to the gym 3 times a week.

This is the most common objection, and it is based on an "all or nothing" fallacy. A 20-minute, high-intensity bodyweight workout at home (push-ups, squats, planks) is infinitely better than doing nothing. The goal is to send a consistent signal to your body. You have time for what you prioritize. This is not about "finding" time; it is about making a strategic investment in your vitality.

I hate running. Do I have to do cardio?

Absolutely not. The best form of cardio is the one you will actually do. If you hate running, do not run. Try cycling, swimming, hiking, a martial arts class, or even just a very brisk walk. The goal is to elevate your heart rate consistently. Find an activity you enjoy, and it will never feel like a chore.

I am not going to give up beer and pizza. Do I have to eat like a monk?

The TIS is about optimization, not deprivation. Follow the 80/20 rule. If 80% of your meals are composed of clean, whole foods (lean proteins, vegetables, healthy fats, complex carbs), then the 20% of the time you enjoy a beer and pizza will have minimal negative impact. It is about your overall lifestyle pattern, not a single meal. The goal is to fuel your body for performance most of the time, so you have the freedom to enjoy life the rest of the time.

These performance drinks sound complicated. Are they really necessary?

Necessary? No. Powerful? Absolutely. You can improve your sexual health through general good nutrition alone. But these drinks are concentrated doses of the specific compounds that directly support blood flow and hormonal health. Think of them as targeted supplements in liquid form. The recipes are in the Appendix for when you are ready to try them.

Commander's Briefing: Chapter 5

- **Your Body is the Chassis for the TIS Engine.** You have a Formula 1 engine. It is useless if the car's body is weak, has flat tires, and runs on poor fuel. Sexual performance is a mental game played in a physical arena. This chapter builds the high-performance chassis.

- **Blood Flow is the Mission's Lifeline (Cardio).** Strong erections are a hydraulic event. Sustained intercourse is an athletic event. Cardio boosts stamina (eliminating the breathlessness barrier), clears the "pipes" for harder erections by increasing Nitric Oxide (NO), and is a natural antidote to the stress hormone cortisol. Aim for 3-4 sessions per week, 120-150 minutes total.

- **Train the Drivetrain, Not Just the Armor (Strength).** Beach muscles are for show; performance muscles are for function. Your true engines are your Hips and Glutes (the power plant for thrust) and your Core (the center of stability). A weak drivetrain means a stalled mission. Squats, Deadlifts, and Planks are your foundation. Aim for 2-3 sessions per week.

- **High-Performance Fuel for a High-Performance Machine (Nutrition).** A world-class engine sputters on dirty fuel. Prioritize tactical nutrients: Nitric Oxide boosters (leafy greens, beets, watermelon) for blood flow, and Testosterone supporters (zinc, healthy fats, quality sleep). See Appendix B: TIS Performance Drinks for concentrated formulas.

- **Eliminate the Saboteurs.** Visceral fat converts testosterone to estrogen through aromatase. Smoking destroys blood vessels. Excessive alcohol depresses your system. Even poor oral health causes systemic inflammation. Know your enemies and eliminate them.

- **Sleep is Non-Negotiable.** Testosterone is manufactured during deep sleep. 7-9 hours of quality sleep is essential equipment maintenance.

- **Three Starting Points, One Destination.** Physical readiness falls into three categories: foundational conditioning (cardiovascular base and basic strength), hormonal optimization (addressing visceral fat and its testosterone-converting effects), and mobility restoration (flexibility and injury prevention). Identify which category demands your attention first and begin there.

CHAPTER 6

THE CHRONOS TACTIC: COMMANDING YOUR TIME, COMMANDING YOUR PRESENCE

The Invisible Thief

THE TEXT CAME FROM John at 11:47 PM on a Tuesday: "Techniques working. Body ready. But I'm so mentally fried by bedtime that I can't access any of it. What am I missing?"

Matt sent a similar message a few days later: "My schedule is chaos. By the time I get home, I'm empty. How do I give her presence when I have nothing left to give?"

David's message was the most telling: "I realized I manage million-dollar construction timelines with military precision. But my home life? Complete chaos. I'm more disciplined with concrete deliveries than with my own family."

Three men. Three variations of the same problem. They had mastered the techniques. They had built their bodies. But an invisible thief was stealing the one resource that made everything else possible: their mental presence.

This chapter is about catching that thief.

The Cult of Presence

For the modern man, "busy" has become more than a description of a full calendar; it is a badge of honor. A synonym for "important," "in-demand," and "successful." We wear our exhaustion like a medal, bragging about how little we slept as if it were a measure of our worth.

But "I do not have time" is not a statement of fact. It is a declaration of surrender.

In Chapter 5, you forged your body into a machine capable of incredible endurance. But a tired, distracted, and chronically rushed mind cannot command even the fittest body. A man who is constantly racing against the clock cannot be fully present with his partner. His body may be in the bedroom, but his mind is in the boardroom, on the next email, on tomorrow's deadline. This is the death of synchronization. A rushed mind creates a rushed body, triggering the very same Fight or Flight response you have worked so hard to tame.

This chapter will teach you to stop seeing time as an enemy to be conquered and start seeing it as a resource to be strategically allocated. This is not about squeezing more tasks into your day. It is the art of life engineering, a system designed to create the mental and emotional bandwidth required for a truly exceptional intimate life. A man who commands his time offers his partner the most valuable gift of all: his undivided attention.

Three Men, Three Journeys

John's Always-On Prison

I understood John's problem the moment I saw his apartment.

He had invited me over to troubleshoot why the techniques were not translating into results. The answer was visible before he said a word: his laptop sat open on the kitchen table, Slack notifications pinging softly in the background. His phone buzzed on the counter. A second monitor on a desk in the corner displayed an endless scroll of emails.

"This is your problem," I said, gesturing at the digital chaos surrounding us.

"What do you mean? I work from home. This is just how it is."

"No," I said. "This is how you've allowed it to be."

Working from home meant work never truly ended. Slack notifications pinged at 9 PM. "Quick" emails arrived at 10 PM. His laptop sat open on the kitchen table, a constant reminder of unfinished tasks. By the time he finally closed it, his girlfriend was already asleep, or they were both too mentally depleted for anything beyond scrolling their phones in silence.

"We live together," John admitted, "but some weeks it felt like we were just roommates who occasionally made eye contact."

His breakthrough came from the *Sunday Mission Briefing*. By time-blocking his deep work hours and setting a hard "laptop closed" rule at 7 PM, he reclaimed his evenings. The boundary felt uncomfortable at first. His anxiety whispered that he was falling behind. But within two weeks, he noticed something remarkable: his work quality improved because his focused hours were truly focused. And his evenings became his own again.

The first Thursday *Connection Night* felt awkward. Scheduled intimacy? It sounded clinical. But by the third week, both he and his girlfriend were looking forward to it. They texted each other during the day about it. The anticipation itself became part of the experience. What had felt like a corporate calendar entry transformed into something they both protected fiercely.

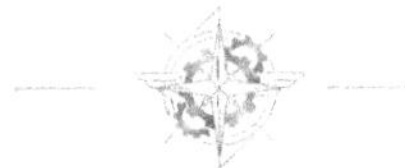

Matt's Unpredictable Schedule

Matt almost dismissed this chapter entirely. "You don't understand," he told me during a school pickup. "My schedule is genuinely unpredictable. I get called in at 2 AM. I can't plan anything."

"What percentage of your time is truly unpredictable?" I asked.

He paused. "I don't know. All of it?"

"Think about it. Your on-call schedule follows a pattern.

Your administrative days are fixed. What's the actual unpredictable portion?"

He was quiet for a moment, doing the math. "Maybe... thirty percent?"

"So seventy percent of your time is predictable, and you've let the thirty percent dominate your perception of the entire hundred."

His expression shifted. Something clicked.

This belief had become his excuse for years.

His wife had stopped expecting him for dinner.

Date nights were a distant memory.

Their intimate life had become a matter of chance: if they both happened to be awake, not exhausted, and in the mood at the same moment, something might happen.

This coincidence occurred perhaps once a month.

He started scheduling Connection Nights on his known off-call evenings, with a backup date built into the following week.

If Tuesday's emergency surgery ran until midnight, Thursday became the protected evening instead.

His wife initially laughed at the formality of it.

"Are we really putting sex on the calendar?"

Six months later, she called it "the best thing we have ever done for our marriage."

Not because of the intimacy itself, though that had improved dramatically.

But because the act of scheduling communicated something she had stopped believing: that she was still his priority.

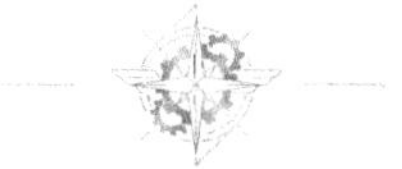

David's Selective Discipline

"Let me get this straight," I said during one of our conversations. "You manage timelines for million-dollar construction projects. Color-coded. Optimized to the hour. Every task tracked, every deadline visible."

"That's my job," he said.

"And at home?"

Silence.

"Complete chaos," he finally admitted. "Evenings bleed into phone calls. Weekends disappear. I haven't had an uninterrupted dinner with my family in... I don't even know how long."

"You apply military discipline to concrete deliveries but not to your daughter's volleyball games."

He winced. "When you put it that way..."

"I'm putting it that way because that's what it is."

The realization hit during his daughter's volleyball game. He was there, technically. He had driven to the school, found a seat in the bleachers, even cheered a few times. But his phone kept buzzing, and he kept glancing at it. Construction emergencies that could not wait. Subcontractor drama that needed immediate attention.

After the game, his daughter ran up to him, excited. "Did you see my serve? The good one? I finally got the rotation right!"

He had not seen it. He had been responding to a text about delayed concrete delivery.

"Which serve?" he asked, trying to cover.

Her face fell. She knew. She always knew.

"Never mind," she said, and walked toward her mother.

That evening, David sat in his home office and stared at his project management software. Every construction task was tracked. Every deadline was visible. His professional life was a model of organized discipline.

He opened a new project. Titled it "Family."

He started blocking time. Hard stops on work calls by 6 PM, three days a week. Weekends became "offline" unless there was a true emergency, and he defined "emergency" strictly: someone in physical danger, not a subcontractor's scheduling conflict.

It felt uncomfortable at first. His phone still buzzed. The urge to check was almost physical. But he remembered the look on his daughter's face and left the phone in his office.

At her next game, he sat in the front row. Phone locked in the car. Eyes on the court.

She served. The rotation was perfect. The ball sailed over the net and landed precisely in the corner.

She looked up at him immediately, searching the bleachers.

He was on his feet, cheering. Their eyes met. She grinned, pumped her fist, and ran back to her position.

After the game, she ran to him again. "You saw it!"

"I saw it," he said. "That was incredible."

She hugged him, hard. He could not remember the last time she had hugged him like that.

His wife watched from a few feet away, her expression unreadable. Later, in the car, she reached over and squeezed his hand.

"You were there today," she said. "Really there."

"I am trying."

"I noticed."

That night, after the kids were in bed, she reached for him. Not out of obligation or routine, but with something that felt like desire. Like he had earned something back.

The irony was not lost on him. He had commanded timelines for million-dollar projects. He had just never applied that same discipline to the only project that truly mattered.

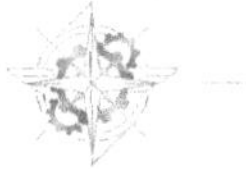

The Time Scarcity Myth: Defining the True Enemy

"I do not have time" is not a fact; it is a feeling. It is a symptom not of a true lack of time, but of a lack of priorities and a flawed strategy. When your mind operates in a constant state of "scarcity," it has profound and destructive effects on your performance, both in and out of the bedroom.

Parkinson's Law states that work expands to fill the time available for its completion. Give yourself a whole day for a three-hour task, and your brain will find ways to make it feel all-consuming. Without clear boundaries and defined objectives, your mental energy dissipates across the vast, unstructured expanse of your day, like a gas expanding to fill any container.

Decision Fatigue is the result of your brain's finite capacity for high-quality decisions being drained by hundreds of unplanned micro-choices throughout the day. *Should I check my email now? What should I work on next? What is for lunch?* By evening, the last thing a fatigued mind wants is to engage in something as nuanced and demanding as deep intimacy. It craves the path of least resistance: passive entertainment or sleep.

The *Zeigarnik Effect* describes how our brains remain fixated on unfinished tasks. An unstructured day filled with half-finished projects and unanswered emails creates a constant, low-grade hum of mental anxiety. Your brain keeps sending notifications about all the open loops. This mental clutter makes true presence impossible.

When you enter the bedroom with a mind in a state of scarcity and fatigue, you have already sabotaged the TIS engine before you have even turned the key. The thought, *I have to hurry because I have an early meeting tomorrow*, triggers the same Fight or Flight panic as performance anxiety.

The purpose of the *Chronos Tactic* is to destroy this scarcity mindset and replace it with one of tactical abundance. You have more than enough time for what matters. You simply need to command it.

Tactic 1: The Mission Briefing (The Sunday Evening Strategy)

A commander does not send his army into battle without a plan. An apex man does not stumble into his week reacting to whatever comes his way. Twenty minutes, just twenty minutes, every Sunday evening can bring the chaos of the next seven days under your absolute control.

Step 1: Conduct a Brain Dump. Get everything out of your head. Use a notebook or a digital document. Write down every single task, personal and professional, that you feel you need to accomplish in the coming week, from "finalize the budget report" to "buy dog food" to "call mom." This act alone reduces the Zeigarnik effect by externalizing your mental to-do list. What lives on paper no longer needs to occupy mental RAM.

Step 2: Identify Your *Big Rocks*. Not all tasks are created equal. As Stephen Covey taught, imagine your week is an empty jar. Your Big Rocks are the 3-5 most important missions that will truly move the needle in your career and life. Everything else is secondary gravel and sand. If you put the sand and gravel in first, the big rocks will never fit. You must place your priorities first.

Step 3: Time-Block Your Calendar. Schedule time blocks for your Big Rocks as if they were unbreakable appointments with your most important client. A mission to "Write the Q3 Report" becomes a concrete, 2-hour block on Tuesday from 9 AM to 11 AM. These hours are now booked. Be ruthless in protecting this time.

Step 4: Schedule Buffer Time. Schedule 30-minute blocks of "buffer" or "flex" time throughout your week. This is for the unexpected calls, the tasks that run long, the fires you have to put out. This prevents a single disruption from derailing your entire day. It is the shock absorber for your week. Without buffer time, one delayed meeting creates a cascade of stress that follows you into the evening.

Step 5: Master the Tactical *No*. When your plan is this clear, it becomes exponentially easier to say *no* to non-essential requests. Your *no* is no longer a vague rejection; it is a strategic decision based on pre-allocated resources. "I cannot do that on Tuesday morning because I am allocated to the Q3 report, but I can look at it on Wednesday during my flex time." A tactical *no* to a low-priority task is a powerful *yes* to your most important goals.

This simple planning ritual eliminates the massive mental drain of uncertainty. You wake up on Monday morning knowing your mission. Your mental energy is no longer wasted on *what should I do?*; it is focused entirely on *how do I execute this with excellence?*

Tactic 2: Deep Work Blocks (The Sniper Approach)

Multitasking is a myth of productivity. What we call multitasking is actually rapid *task-switching*. Every time you switch, from your report, to your email, to a text message, and back, your brain pays a cognitive tax. Research shows that each switch leaves *attention residue*, a portion of your mind still processing the previous task. It is like using a shotgun, firing randomly in all directions and hoping you hit something. The result is shallow work, drained energy, and a feeling of being busy but not productive.

Instead, a commander adopts the Sniper Approach. One target. One shot. Total focus.

Step 1: Define the Mission. Choose one, and only one, important task from your Big Rocks list.

Step 2: Set the Timer. Dedicate an uninterrupted 60 or 90-minute block of time to this task. Use a physical timer or a dedicated app, not your phone's timer which is a gateway to distraction.

Step 3: Go Dark (*The Digital Fortress*). This is non-negotiable. Create what pilots call a *sterile cockpit*, an environment free of all non-essential distractions. Turn off all notifications on your computer. Not "vibrate." Off. Close your email tab entirely. Do not minimize it. Close it. Put your phone in another room. If this feels extreme, that feeling itself reveals how dependent your brain has become on the dopamine of notifications. If you work in an open office, use noise-canceling headphones as a signal that you are unavailable.

The goal is to create an environment where distraction is not merely resisted but made impossible. Willpower is a finite resource. Do not waste it fighting your phone when you could simply remove it from the equation.

Step 4: Execute. Direct all your mental energy toward that single target. If your mind wanders, gently guide it back to the mission, just as you would during meditation. This is not a failure; it is the training itself.

The Transfer Effect

As you build this "deep focus" muscle in your professional life, you will carry the same ability into your intimate life. The skill is transferable. A mind trained to ignore the pull of a smartphone notification can also ignore the pull of a work worry during intimate moments. When you are with your partner, your mind will no longer be reflexively reaching for the distraction of a phone or ruminating on a work problem. Your only target at that moment is the sensory experience of being with your partner. This is undivided attention in its purest, most powerful form.

Tactic 3: Scheduling Intimacy (The Priority Target)

The thought, *You cannot schedule sex, that is so unromantic!* is the most common objection to this approach. It is a romanticized fantasy from movies that great intimacy should just *happen* spontaneously after a long, stressful day. For busy, successful adults with careers, children, and commitments, this is a recipe for a sexless relationship.

The reality is this: What gets scheduled, gets done. You schedule dentist appointments. You schedule meetings with your team. You schedule your workouts. You schedule these things because they are important. Is your intimate connection with your partner not at least as important?

Scheduling intimacy is not about making it a clinical, passionless chore. It is the ultimate act of romance. It is the difference between saying, "Maybe we will have sex if I have any energy left at the end of the day," and declaring, "I have reserved and protected a specific time for us this week, and I will let nothing interrupt it because you are my priority." The planning does not kill the romance; the planning is what enables the romance to happen.

Step 1: Mark the Calendar. In your weekly mission briefing, mark one or two evenings a week in your calendar as Connection Night or any code name you and your partner choose. This is now a Big Rock. Treat it with the same sanctity as a board meeting.

Step 2: Set the Rules of Engagement. This is a period of time where phones are turned off, laptops are closed, and you are focused only on each other. The outside world ceases to exist for this block of time.

Step 3: Remove the Goal. A Connection Night does not necessarily have to lead to sex. The only goal is connection. Sometimes this will lead to a deep conversation over a glass of wine, other times to a massage, and other times to a passionate night. By removing the pressure of a specific outcome, you create the space for genuine desire to emerge.

Communicating With Your Partner

Frame it as a solution to a shared problem, not as something you are imposing. Consider language like this:
"I have been thinking about us lately. We have both been so busy and stressed, and I hate that it leaves us with no energy for each other at the end of the day. What if we protected some time for ourselves? We could block out Thursday evening as 'our night,' no phones, no work, just us. What we do with that time is completely up to us in the moment."

This approach acknowledges a shared struggle rather than assigning blame. It positions you as proactive and invested in the relationship. It invites collaboration rather than dictating terms. And it removes performance pressure by leaving the outcome open.

A partner who feels like a priority enters the bedroom with an energy of openness, safety, and desire. A partner who feels like an afterthought, squeezed in between emails and exhaustion, enters with resentment and disconnection.

The Bookends: Morning and Evening Rituals

The way you start and end your day creates the container for everything in between.

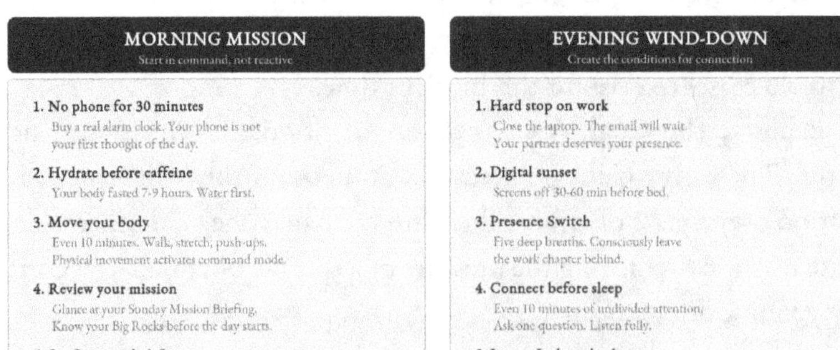

A proactive morning builds command. A proper evening builds connection.

These "bookends" determine whether you enter the bedroom as a depleted, scattered man or as a calm, present commander.

The Morning Launch Sequence

A reactive morning, immediately checking emails and social media, puts you on the defensive from the moment you wake. A proactive morning puts you in command.

The TIS Morning Protocol:

No phone for the first 30 minutes. Your phone is not an alarm clock. Buy a real alarm clock. The moment you check your phone, you surrender your mental agenda to whoever sent you notifications overnight.

Hydrate before you caffeinate. Your body has been fasting for 7-9 hours. A large glass of water with lemon starts your system correctly.

Move your body. Even 10 minutes of stretching, a short walk, or basic calisthenics activates your physiology and clears mental fog.

Review your mission. Spend 5 minutes with your calendar. Know your Big Rocks for the day. Visualize successful completion.

Protect your peak hours. Schedule your most demanding cognitive work for your first 3-4 hours. This is when your decision-making capacity is highest.

A man who owns his morning owns his day. A man who owns his day arrives home with reserves rather than deficits.

The Evening Wind-Down Protocol

Remember the Recovery Factor from Chapter 5? Quality sleep is essential for testosterone production and overall vitality. But you cannot simply collapse into bed after staring at screens and expect restorative sleep. Your nervous system needs a transition period.

The TIS Evening Protocol:

Hard stop on work. Choose a time, whether 6 PM, 7 PM, or 8 PM, and make it non-negotiable. When that time arrives, work stops. Laptop closes.

Digital sunset. One hour before bed, screens go off or switch to night mode. The blue light from devices suppresses melatonin production and signals to your brain that it is still daytime.

Transition ritual. A shower, light stretching, reading a physical book, or a brief conversation with your partner about the day. The specific activity matters less than the consistency. Your brain learns to associate this ritual with the transition to rest.

Bedroom environment. Cool temperature (65-68°F / 18-20°C), complete darkness, no screens. Your bedroom should be associated with only two activities: sleep and intimacy.

Connection before sleep. Even on non-scheduled nights, five minutes of undistracted conversation or physical touch with your partner maintains the bond. This does not need to lead anywhere. It simply reinforces that you end the day together, not separately scrolling your phones.

This evening protocol ensures the quality sleep your body needs for hormonal health and creates natural opportunities for connection that a chaotic, screen-dominated evening destroys.

For the Connection Night Planning Guide and Money Date Template, see Appendix F: The Connection Toolkit. For digital tools designed to support your time management and scheduling practice tismethod.com/tactical-intimacy/book-owners or see Appendix A: TIS Digital Resources.

Commander's Q&A: Time and Intimacy

This all sounds great, but my job is genuinely unpredictable. I cannot always stick to a schedule.

The goal of a plan is not rigidity; it is to provide a default to return to. A ship's captain has a course plotted, but he is always ready to adjust for a storm. If an emergency torpedoes your Tuesday morning deep work block, your weekly plan allows you to quickly assess and move it to your Wednesday flex time without losing momentum. Focus on what you can control. Build flexibility into the system with buffer time and backup dates. The plan is your map. Even if you have to take a detour, you still know where you are going, which prevents the feeling of being lost and overwhelmed.

Will scheduling intimacy not kill the spontaneity and passion?

It is a myth that spontaneity is the source of passion. The true source of passion is desire, and desire thrives on anticipation and priority. Knowing that "Thursday night is our night" allows for a slow burn of anticipation to build throughout the day for both of you. It gives you something to look forward to, to text about, to mentally prepare for. You can build tension and excitement leading up to your scheduled time. This is far more romantic than the alternative, which is often two exhausted people scrolling on their phones in bed, vaguely hoping something might happen before one of them falls asleep. That is not spontaneity. That is neglect disguised as flexibility.

How do I explain the "no phone in the morning" rule to colleagues who expect immediate responses?

You train people how to treat you. If you have historically responded to emails within minutes at all hours, you have trained your colleagues to expect that. Retraining takes time but is entirely possible. Start by delaying your responses slightly. If you typically respond at 6:30 AM, respond at 8 AM instead. Within a few weeks, people adjust their expectations. For truly urgent matters, colleagues can call. But you will likely discover that almost nothing is as urgent as the sender believes it to be. Your morning mental clarity is worth more than the minor convenience of instant responses. Protect it accordingly.

My partner is resistant to the idea of scheduled intimacy. How do I proceed?

Do not push. The worst thing you can do is make your partner feel pressured or scheduled *at* rather than *with*. Instead, focus on what you can control unilaterally: your own time management, your presence when you are together, your evening wind-down routine. As your partner experiences you as more present, more calm, and more attentive, they may become more open to discussing structured time together. You might also start smaller. Rather than scheduling intimacy directly, schedule *unplugged time* with no agenda. A weekly evening where phones go away and you simply spend time together. Let the intimacy emerge naturally from that protected space. Once your partner experiences the value of that protected time, the conversation about expanding it becomes much easier.

Commander's Briefing: Chapter 6

- **Time is Not Your Enemy; Your Perception of It Is.** "I am busy" is not a badge of honor; it is a surrender of your potential. A rushed mind creates a rushed body, triggering the Fight or Flight response. Commanding your time creates the most valuable gift you can offer your partner: your undivided attention.

- **Destroy the Scarcity Mindset.** "I do not have time" is not a fact; it is a feeling. It stems from Parkinson's Law (work expands to fill available time), Decision Fatigue (depleted willpower from unplanned micro-choices), and the Zeigarnik Effect (mental fixation on unfinished tasks). Structure eliminates all three.

- **Tactic 1: The Sunday Evening Mission Briefing.** Twenty minutes on a Sunday evening allows you to command your week. Brain dump every task, identify your 3-5 Big Rocks, time-block them in your calendar, schedule buffer time for the unexpected, and master the tactical "no."

- **Tactic 2: Adopt the Sniper Approach (Deep Work).** Multitasking is rapid task-switching that creates a cognitive tax. Instead: one target, one shot, total focus. Create a Digital Fortress, eliminate all distractions, and direct your full attention to a single mission. This skill transfers directly to your intimate life.

- **Tactic 3: Schedule Intimacy as a Priority Target.** What gets scheduled, gets done. Scheduling intimacy is not clinical; it is the ultimate act of romance. It declares "you are my priority." Frame it as a solution to a shared problem, invite collaboration, and remove outcome pressure.

- **Master the Bookends.** A proactive morning (no phone for 30 minutes, hydrate, move, review your mission) puts you in command. A proper evening wind-down (hard stop on work, digital sunset, transition ritual) ensures quality sleep and creates natural opportunities for connection.

- **Three Variations, One Solution.** Time management failures fall into three patterns: the always-on trap (no boundary between work and personal life), the unpredictability illusion (letting a small percentage of chaos dominate your perception of the whole), and selective discipline (applying professional rigor everywhere except where it matters most). Identify your pattern and address it directly.

Chapter 7

The Abundance Tactic: Commanding Your Finances, Commanding Your Confidence

The Ghost That Followed Them Home

I NOTICED SOMETHING TROUBLING as John, Matt, and David progressed through their journeys.

Their techniques were solid. Their bodies were transforming. Their time management was improving. Yet all three still carried a tension I could see in their shoulders, hear in their voices, feel in the way they deflected certain questions.

It was John who finally named it. We were talking over the fence one evening when his girlfriend called from inside, something about a restaurant reservation.

"We can't," he called back. Then, quieter, to me: "I'm making more money than I ever have. Why do I feel broker than ever?"

Matt admitted something similar during a school pickup. "I earn more in a month than my father earned in a year. But I lie awake at 2 AM doing math in my head. How is that possible?"

David's version was different but familiar. "Some months I feel like a king. Other months I snap at my wife over a grocery bill. She never knows which version of me she's going to get."

Three men. Three income levels. The same ghost haunting all of them: financial stress. And that ghost was following them into the bedroom.

Financial stress is one of the most powerful libido killers known to science. When your brain perceives financial threat, it activates the same Fight or Flight response we have been working to control. Cortisol floods your system. Testosterone drops. Your body literally deprioritizes reproduction because it perceives that survival is at stake. Money consistently ranks among the top sources of significant stress for men, and financial disagreements are among the strongest predictors of divorce, outranking conflicts about children, household responsibilities, and even infidelity. The stress does not stay contained in spreadsheets and bank statements. It bleeds into every conversation, every decision, every moment of intimacy.

Financial anxiety occupies the same mental bandwidth that presence requires. A man cannot calculate interest rates and be emotionally available at the same time. This mental burden triggers the same survival response you have worked so hard to tame, making relaxation and deep connection a biological impossibility.

Conversely, financial control is one of the most powerful and underrated forms of confidence. A man who commands his money, who has a clear plan and looks to the future with certainty, carries himself differently. This confidence is reflected in his posture, in the calm cadence of his speech, and in the grounded, stable energy he projects. He offers his partner genuine stability and security. This is not about being rich. It is about being in command. Your partner does not feel safe because of the number in your bank account; she feels safe because you are calmly steering the ship.

This chapter gives you the tools to eliminate financial stress as a saboteur of your intimate life.

Three Men, Three Financial Journeys

John's Lifestyle Inflation Trap

John's financial awakening started with a question I asked him over the fence.

"Your salary doubled in three years," I said. "How much more are you saving now compared to before?"

He paused. Thought about it. His face changed.

"The same," he admitted. "Maybe less."

"Where did the money go?"

He started listing: the nicer apartment, the newer car, the premium subscriptions, the meal delivery service he kept forgetting to cancel. With each item, his voice got quieter.

"I upgraded everything except my security," he said finally. "I'm on a treadmill."

Every raise had come with an upgrade. A nicer apartment in a trendier neighborhood. A newer car with a higher monthly payment. Premium subscriptions to services he barely used. His income grew, but his savings stayed flat. And with no emergency fund, every unexpected expense triggered the same old anxiety.

His girlfriend noticed. "You make good money," she said one evening after he snapped at her over a restaurant bill. "Why are you always stressed about it?"

The question stung because he had no good answer. The stress followed him everywhere, including into the bedroom. On nights when he should have been present with her, his mind was running calculations, wondering how he would cover next month's credit card bill.

John's breakthrough came when he tracked every expense for 30 days and discovered he was spending over $800 monthly on subscriptions and services he barely valued. Within three months of cutting the waste and automating savings, he had his first real emergency fund. He stopped snapping. He stopped calculating during dinner. He started being present.

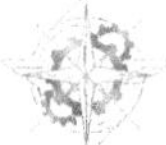

Matt's High Income Trap

The conversation with Matt happened in the school parking lot, both of us waiting for our kids.

"Can I ask you something personal?" he said, staring at his phone without really seeing it.

"Of course."

"Do you ever feel like you're earning a lot but building nothing?"

I let the question sit. He needed to say more.

"I deserve things," he continued. "After the shifts I work, the decisions I make, the lives I hold in my hands. I deserve the watch, the car, the weekend getaways. That's what I tell myself. But my wife sees the bank statements. And she sees something different."

"What does she see?"

"A man who earns a fortune and saves nothing. A high income, not wealth." He finally looked at me. "She doesn't feel secure. And honestly? Neither do I."

After brutal 14-hour shifts in the trauma unit, spending had become his stress relief, his reward for surviving another week of life-and-death decisions. His wife, who managed their household finances, saw a different picture: high income, minimal savings, and a lifestyle that would collapse if he ever stopped working.

"We earn a lot," she finally said after another argument about an impulse purchase, "but we are not building anything."

The distinction hit him hard. Income is what you earn. Wealth is what you keep. A high earner has cash flow. A wealthy person has options. Matt had no options. If he stopped working tomorrow, their lifestyle would evaporate within months.

He stopped asking *Can I afford this?* and started asking *Does this build wealth or destroy it?* Within a year, they had eliminated debt and built a substantial emergency fund. His wife noticed the shift before he did. "You seem lighter," she said. "Like you are not carrying something heavy anymore." That lightness followed him into the bedroom.

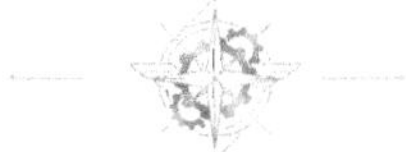

David's Variable Income Reality

David called me during a slow quarter, his voice tight with stress.

"I'm a different person when work is slow," he said. "I know it. My wife knows it. The kids probably know it too. I snap over nothing. I lie awake doing worst-case math. I'm physically home but mentally somewhere else entirely."

"What's the fear?" I asked.

"That the next project won't come. That we'll burn through savings. That I'll have to tell her we need to cut back." He paused. "I manage million-dollar construction budgets. I should be able to manage my own household. But when income is unpredictable, everything feels unpredictable."

"Have you built a buffer?"

Silence. Then: "No. When money comes in, I think we're fine. When it doesn't, I panic. There's no middle ground."

"That's the problem," I said. "You're letting your income volatility become your emotional volatility. Your family is living on your financial roller coaster."

His transformation began with the emergency fund. Six months of expenses felt like climbing Everest, so he started smaller: one month. Then two. Then three.

The next slow quarter still happened, but it no longer triggered panic. He had a buffer. For the first time, he could weather uncertainty without his family bearing the emotional cost. His wife noticed immediately. "You are still you," she said during a lean month. "Even when work is slow, you are still here with us."

That presence extended to the bedroom. Without the constant financial anxiety, he could finally focus on her instead of on spreadsheets.

All three men learned the same lesson: Financial stress does not stay in your bank account. It follows you into every room of your life, including the bedroom. And financial control does not require a specific income level. It requires a system and a mindset.

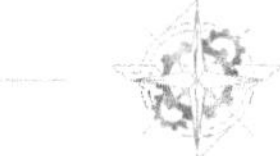

The Scarcity Mindset: Your Brain is Wired to Fear Loss

The source of financial stress is often not the absolute amount of money in your bank account, but your mindset towards it. The scarcity mindset lives in a constant, low-grade fear of "not enough." It turns every financial decision, big or small, into a source of anxiety.

Nobel Prize-winning psychologist Daniel Kahneman explained why with his theory of *Loss Aversion*. His research showed that for the human brain, the psychological pain of losing \$100 is roughly twice as powerful as the pleasure of gaining \$100. Your brain is hardwired to protect what you have far more fiercely than it is to risk it for a potential gain.

This ancient wiring, while useful on the savanna where losing your food supply could mean death, is a disaster in the modern financial world. It keeps you perpetually on the defensive, preventing you from taking calculated risks that lead to growth, and swings you between anxious hoarding (never enjoying your money) and impulsive *what the hell* spending as a form of stress relief (sabotaging your future). It is a cycle of fear and regret.

In the bedroom, this scarcity mindset translates directly into the fear of *not being good enough* or *not having enough* stamina or control. The mental patterns are identical. The first step of the *Abundance Tactic* is to break this programming by seizing control of the data.

The Critical Distinction: Income vs. Wealth

Before we move to tactics, we must address a fundamental misconception that traps many successful men.

Income is what you earn. Wealth is what you keep.

A man earning $300,000 per year who spends $310,000 is poorer than a man earning $60,000 who spends $50,000. The first man is running on a treadmill, dependent on his next paycheck. The second man is building something.

This distinction matters for your intimate life because your partner does not feel secure based on your income. She feels secure based on your financial trajectory. Are you building? Or are you just spending?

The Lifestyle Inflation Trap. Every raise, every bonus, every promotion comes with a temptation: upgrade your lifestyle to match your new income. The antidote is simple but counterintuitive: When your income increases, increase your savings rate, not your spending. A man who earns $100,000 and saves $20,000 is in a stronger position than a man who earns $200,000 and saves $20,000. The first man has learned to live below his means. The second man is one unexpected expense away from crisis.

Tactic 1: Map the Battlefield (Know Your Numbers)

A commander does not go into battle without a detailed map of the terrain. You cannot achieve financial freedom without a clear, brutally honest picture of your financial situation. The stress of uncertainty is always a hundred times worse than the stress of a hard truth. Clarity is control.

Step 1: Calculate Your Net Income. This is your take-home pay after taxes. Know this number to the dollar. This is your total available ammunition for the month.

Step 2: Track Every Single Expense. For one full month, track every cent you spend. Use a simple notebook or a budgeting app like Mint, YNAB (You Need A Budget), or Personal Capital. Be ruthless. That $5 coffee, that unplanned lunch, that impulse online purchase, it all goes on the list. This is not about judging yourself; it is about gathering intelligence. You are a data analyst, not a defendant.

Step 3: Analyze the Data. At the end of the month, categorize your spending. Look at the numbers without judgment, as a race engineer would look at telemetry data. Where is the money really going? Which expenses are fixed (rent, car payment), and which are variable (dining out, entertainment)? Ask yourself three critical questions: **The Value Question:** Which of these purchases brought me genuine, lasting value or joy? **The Alignment Question:** Does this spending pattern align with the man I want to be and the life I want to build? **The Leakage Question:** Where is the mindless spending on things I do not truly value that could be redirected to my goals?

Step 4: Implement the 50/30/20 Rule. As a starting framework, allocate 50% of your net income to Needs (housing, utilities, groceries), 30% to Wants (hobbies, travel, dining out), and 20% to Savings and Debt Repayment. This is not a rigid law, but a powerful diagnostic tool to see where your spending is out of alignment.

The 50/30/20 Framework

This simple act of tracking and analyzing is profoundly empowering. You are no longer in the dark, haunted by a vague sense of financial dread. You have the map. You are in control.

A man who knows his numbers sleeps better. He does not lie awake at 2 AM running calculations. When the lights go out, his mind is clear. When his partner reaches for him, he is present, not mentally reviewing bank statements.

Tactic 2: Build Your Fortress (The Emergency Fund)

The greatest trigger for acute financial stress is the unexpected: a car breakdown, a sudden health issue, an unexpected job loss. An emergency fund is your fortress. It is the armor that allows you to withstand life's blows without flinching. It is the ultimate "sleep well at night" account, your personal bailout fund that severs the link between an unexpected event and a financial crisis.

The Goal: Save enough money to cover 3 to 6 months of essential living expenses (rent, bills, food, your "Needs" from the 50/30/20 rule) in a separate, high-yield savings account. This money is not for investments. It is not for a vacation. It is a sacred fund that you do not touch except in a true emergency.

The Start: Do not let the final goal intimidate you. Start with $100 today. Set up an automatic transfer from your checking account to your emergency fund savings account for a small, manageable amount every week or every paycheck.

The key is automation and consistency. Pay yourself first, before any other discretionary spending.

The Result: As this fund grows, you will feel a deep sense of psychological relief that money cannot buy. It is the quiet confidence of knowing that you have built a wall between you and the chaos of the world.

David's story illustrates this perfectly. His variable income meant that without an emergency fund, every slow quarter triggered survival mode. His body remained at home, but his nervous system was in crisis. With six months of expenses in reserve, a slow quarter became an inconvenience, not an emergency. The emergency fund did not just protect his finances. It protected his presence. It protected his relationship. It protected his intimate life.

Tactic 3: The Attack Plan (Building an Abundance Mindset)

Once your fortress is built and your budget is clear, it is time to go on the offensive. This is the crucial mental shift from a defensive scarcity mindset to an offensive abundance mindset.

See Money as a Tool, Not a Scorecard. Money is not a measure of your worth; it is a tool to build the life you desire. A scarcity mindset hoards money out of fear. An abundance mindset deploys money strategically to create value and experiences. Money spent on experiences (a trip, a memorable dinner with your partner) or growth (a course, a book, a gym membership) provides far more lasting happiness than materialistic spending that provides only a momentary high. An experience becomes a part of who you are; a material object is just something you own.

Practice Value-Based Spending. Before making a non-essential purchase over a certain amount (say, $50), implement a mandatory 24-hour waiting period. After 24 hours, ask yourself: *What will this truly add to my life? Does this align with my long-term goals and values?* This simple question acts as a powerful filter against impulsive, dopamine-driven purchases and trains you to spend with intention.

Invest in Yourself (Your Greatest Asset). Your greatest asset is not your bank account; it is your ability to earn, to learn, and to grow. Money spent on learning a new skill, improving your health, or developing your mind will pay you back exponentially for the rest of your life. A man with an abundance mindset knows that the best investment he can ever make is in himself, because he is the engine of his own wealth creation.

A man who feels this confidence enters the bedroom without financial baggage, carrying only the desire for pleasure and connection. He does not need to prove anything. He does not need to compensate for insecurity with performance. He is simply present, confident, and generous.

The Money Date: Financial Alignment With Your Partner

In Chapter 4, you learned the importance of enlisting your partner as a co-pilot. Financial alignment is perhaps the most critical area for this partnership.

Financial disagreements are among the strongest predictors of divorce. This is not because money itself is so important, but because money represents values, priorities, security, and trust. When partners are misaligned financially, they are misaligned on a fundamental level.

The solution is the *Money Date*, a scheduled, regular conversation about finances that prevents small misalignments from becoming relationship-destroying conflicts.

How to Implement the Money Date

Frequency: Monthly, scheduled like any important appointment.

Format: A relaxed setting, perhaps over coffee or wine. This is not a confrontation; it is a partnership meeting.

Agenda: Review the past month: what did you spend, where did you succeed, where did you slip? Discuss upcoming expenses and any large purchases on the horizon. Check progress on shared goals: emergency fund, debt payoff, vacation savings. Align on values: are there any spending patterns you want to change, any investments in your relationship or growth you want to make?

Tone: Approach this with the same Soft Start-Up you learned in Chapter 4. This is "us versus the problem," not "me versus you."

Rules: No blame for past spending; the goal is forward progress, not relitigating history. No major financial decisions made in the moment; discuss, then decide later. Both partners have equal voice, regardless of who earns more.

A couple that is financially aligned is a couple that trusts each other. They are rowing in the same direction. The tension that comes from hidden spending, conflicting priorities, or unspoken resentments dissolves. When you know you and your partner are building together, when there are no financial secrets simmering beneath the surface, you can be fully vulnerable with each other. Financial transparency creates emotional safety. Emotional safety creates the conditions for exceptional intimacy.

All three men eventually implemented some version of the Money Date. John and his girlfriend started with weekly check-ins, given how much financial ground they needed to cover. "It felt weird at first," John admitted. "Talking about money like it was a project. But now it's just part of us. We're building something together instead of just spending together."

Matt's Money Dates became monthly rituals. His wife went from critic to partner. "She's not worried about my spending anymore," he told me. "Because she sees the plan. She's part of the plan."

David and his wife used their Money Dates to create what he called "the buffer conversation," a monthly check on their emergency fund and a shared understanding of where they stood. "Even during slow quarters," David said, "we're calm. Because we both know the numbers. We both know we're okay."

For the Money Date Template and planning guide, see Appendix F: The Connection Toolkit. For digital tools, visit tismethod.com/tactical-intimacy/book-o wners

Commander's Q&A: Financial Operations

My partner and I have very different views on money. How do I even start this conversation?

Approach it just like the conversation in Chapter 4: with a Soft Start-Up and a "we" focus. Frame it as a team project to build a shared future. Say something like, "I would love for us to build a financial plan together, not because we are in trouble, but because I want us to be a powerful team working towards our shared dreams, like traveling or buying a house. I want us to feel completely in control of our future together." Start with shared goals before addressing areas of conflict. Find common ground first.

I am overwhelmed by debt. An emergency fund feels impossible.

When you are in a hole, the first step is to stop digging. The "Map the Battlefield" tactic is even more critical for you. Once you see exactly where your money is going, you can identify areas to cut back and redirect that cash flow towards paying down your highest-interest debt first (this is called the "debt avalanche" method for the fastest mathematical path to being debt-free). For a psychological boost, you could also try the "debt snowball" method: pay off your smallest debt first, regardless of interest rate, to get a quick win and build momentum. Even a tiny emergency fund of $500 can be a huge psychological relief while you tackle your debt, acting as a buffer against further debt. Do not wait until you are debt-free to start building security. Build both simultaneously, even if the amounts are small.

Investing seems complicated and risky. Is it not just gambling?

Day-trading based on hot tips can be gambling. However, a disciplined, long-term strategy of investing in low-cost index funds (which hold a small piece of hundreds of the largest companies, like the S&P 500) is one of the most reliable and proven ways to build wealth over time. It is the difference between betting on a single horse and owning a small piece of every horse in the race. The abundance mindset is not about getting rich quick; it is about making consistent, intelligent decisions that allow your money to work for you over the long run. The goal is not to beat the market; it is to be the market.

How do I talk to my partner about spending habits without it turning into a fight?

Focus on shared goals, not individual behavior. Instead of "You spend too much on clothes," try "I want us to save for a vacation together. Can we look at our spending and see where we can find room for that?" Make it about building toward something positive, not restricting behavior. No one wants to feel controlled. Everyone wants to feel like they are working toward a dream. The Money Date framework helps because it creates a regular, neutral space for these conversations. When financial discussions are scheduled and expected, they feel less like ambushes and more like collaboration.

Commander's Briefing: Chapter 7

- **Financial Stress is the Ghost in the Room.** It raises cortisol, triggers your survival response, and makes deep connection a biological impossibility. Financial disagreements are among the strongest predictors of divorce. The stress does not stay in your bank account; it follows you into every room, including the bedroom.

- **Financial Control is Confidence.** This is not about being rich; it is about being in command. A man with a clear financial plan projects stability and security. Your partner feels safe not because of the number in your bank account, but because you are calmly executing a plan.

- **Income is Not Wealth.** A high earner who spends everything is poorer than a moderate earner who saves. Beware lifestyle inflation: when income rises, increase savings, not spending. Ask "Does this build wealth or destroy it?" before every significant purchase.

- **The Enemy is the Scarcity Mindset.** Your brain is wired for loss aversion: losing $100 hurts twice as much as gaining $100 feels good. This ancient programming keeps you oscillating between anxious hoarding and impulsive spending. Break the cycle with data and systems.

- **Tactic 1: Map the Battlefield.** Track every expense for 30 days. The stress of uncertainty is always worse than a hard truth. Apply the 50/30/20 framework (50% Needs, 30% Wants, 20% Savings/Debt). Clarity is control, and control follows you into the bedroom.

- **Tactic 2: Build Your Fortress.** An emergency fund of 3-6 months of essential expenses severs the link between unexpected events and financial crisis. Start small, automate, and build consistently. This is the "sleep well at night" account that protects your presence with your partner.

- **Tactic 3: Go on the Offensive.** Shift from scarcity to abundance. See money as a tool, not a scorecard. Practice value-based spending with a 24-hour rule. Invest in yourself as your greatest asset.

- **The Money Date Creates Alignment.** Monthly financial conversations with your partner, using Soft Start-Up techniques from Chapter 4, prevent small misalignments from becoming conflicts. Financial transparency creates emotional safety. Emotional safety creates the conditions for exceptional intimacy.

- **Three Income Levels, One Solution.** Financial stress wears three common masks: lifestyle inflation (income rises but security stays flat), the high-income trap (earning much but building nothing), and variable income volatility (letting unpredictable cash flow become unpredictable emotions). The solution is identical regardless of income level: map your battlefield, build your fortress, and align with your partner.

CHAPTER 8

THE CHARISMA TACTIC: PROJECTING YOUR POWER, CREATING CONNECTION

The Missing Bridge

SOMETHING WAS NOT ADDING up.

John, Matt, and David had made remarkable progress. Their techniques were solid. Their bodies were transforming. Their time was managed. Their finances were under control. Yet when I checked in with each of them, I heard variations of the same frustration.

"I've done everything right," John said. "But she still says I'm *hard to read*. I don't know how to show her what's inside."

Matt's version: "At work, people hang on my every word. At home, my wife says I'm *not really there*. How can I be so present in the OR and so absent in my own living room?"

David put it most bluntly: "I give my best self to clients and crews. My wife gets whatever's left over. She finally told me: 'Everyone else gets the real David. I get the scraps.'"

Three men with internal power they could not project. Three relationships suffering not from lack of love, but from lack of connection. Three bridges that had never been built.

Picture a high-stakes business meeting. Two men present nearly identical proposals, backed by the same solid data. Robert is brilliant. His slides are packed with information, his logic is flawless, but his voice is monotone and rushed. He nervously shuffles his papers, his eyes darting around the room. James presents his case with the same solid data, but he tells a story with it. He moves with calm, deliberate confidence. His voice is resonant and clear, pausing at key moments to let his points land. He makes sustained eye contact with each person at the table.

Who gets the deal? Every single time, it is James. The difference is not in the content; it is in the delivery. The difference is charisma.

You have mastered your body like an athlete, your time like a commander, and your finances like a strategist. But even the strongest fortress is isolated without bridges connecting it to the outside world. Charisma is your bridge. It is the art that projects your internal power into compelling words, confident touches, and meaningful glances that create deep, authentic connection.

Great sex begins long before you enter the bedroom. It is ignited by an intriguing text message during the day. It is kindled by a deep conversation over dinner. It is stoked by a smoldering look from across the room. Your partner's desire often builds throughout the day, influenced by how seen she felt, how heard she felt, how desired she felt in the hours before. Every interaction is either building that desire or diminishing it. There is no neutral.

Charisma is not a magical gift you are born with. Like every other component of the *Tactical Intimacy System*, it is a set of learnable, practicable, and masterable tactics. This chapter will teach you those tactics.

Three Men, Three Charisma Journeys

John's Introvert Advantage

John almost gave up on this chapter entirely.

"I'm an introvert," he told me over the fence one evening. "This charisma stuff isn't for people like me. I can't be the life of the party. I don't have witty things to say. I just... listen."

"That's exactly the point," I said.

He looked confused.

"John, charisma isn't about talking more. It's about attention quality. And introverts are often better at that than extroverts. You don't need to become someone else. You need to become a more intentional version of who you already are."

He was skeptical. But he agreed to try one thing: putting his phone in another room during dinner conversations. Not on the table. Not in his pocket. In another room entirely.

The breakthrough came when he stopped trying to be more talkative and started being more present. He practiced the detective approach: instead of waiting for his turn to speak, he focused completely on understanding what she was actually saying, the emotions beneath the words.

The first time he used reflective listening, his girlfriend paused mid-sentence. "You actually heard me," she said, surprised. "Like, really heard me."

John discovered that charisma was not about talking more. It was about listening better. His introversion, which he had always seen as a weakness, became his greatest strength. He did not need to fill silences with chatter. He needed to fill them with attention.

The change extended to the bedroom. His girlfriend began initiating more frequently. "I feel closer to you now," she explained. "When we talk, I feel like you actually see me. That makes me want you."

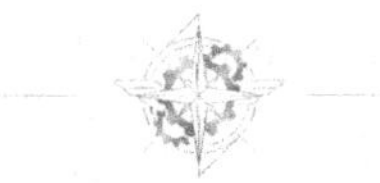

Matt's Presence Switch

I watched the paradox of Matt's life unfold during a school event. He interacted with other parents, teachers, administrators. Attentive.

Engaged. He was magnetic. People gravitated toward him. He remembered names, asked follow-up questions, made everyone feel valued.

Then his wife walked over, and something shifted. His posture changed. His eye contact became intermittent. He answered her question about dinner plans while clearly thinking about something else.

Later, I asked him about it.

"I don't know," he admitted. "At work, I'm 'on.' I have to be. Lives depend on it. But home is where I recover. Where I don't have to perform."

"But you're not recovering," I pointed out. "You're just absent. And your wife isn't getting the man everyone else gets."

He was quiet for a long moment. "She said something like that recently. That I give everyone else my best and give her whatever's left."

His wife received a man who had already spent his best attention on strangers. She felt the absence. "You are here but you are not here," she said one evening. "It is like talking to a ghost."

Matt implemented what he called the *Presence Switch*, a deliberate ritual during his commute home.

He would park in the driveway, take five deep breaths, and consciously tell himself: "Work is complete. That chapter is closed. Home begins now." He visualized leaving the hospital stress in the car.

The change was immediate.

His wife noticed within days. "You are actually looking at me when I talk," she observed. "It is like you are finally home."

That presence transformed their intimate life. His wife no longer felt like she was competing with his job for attention. She had him, all of him, when he walked through that door.

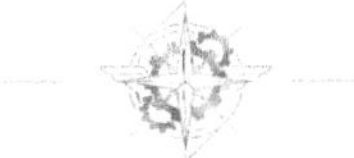

David's Two Versions

David's wife said something to him that he repeated to me, word for word, because he could not stop thinking about it.

"You give everyone else the best of you. I get the scraps."

He called me the next day, shaken. "She's right. I know she's right. But I don't know how to fix it."

"Tell me about work David," I said.

"What do you mean?"

"The guy who walks onto job sites. The one crews respect. The one clients trust. What does that guy do?"

David thought about it. "I remember names. I ask about families. I make eye contact. I'm fully there."

"And home David?"

Silence. Then: "I grunt. I stare at my phone. I'm physically present and mentally gone."

"So you already know how to be charismatic. You just don't do it where it matters most."

The realization hit him hard. Charisma is not a tank that empties. It is a muscle that strengthens with use. And he had been exercising it everywhere except home.

He started applying the same intentional behaviors he used at work: sustained eye contact during conversations, active listening, genuine curiosity about her day, small touches as he passed by. He gave his wife the same quality of attention he gave his most valued professional relationships.

"It is like dating you again," his wife said after a few weeks. The man she had fallen in love with had finally come home.

All three men learned the same lesson: Charisma is not a personality trait. It is a choice. And that choice must be made deliberately, especially with the people who matter most.

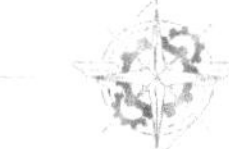

The Foundation of Charisma: The Power of Presence

Everything you have learned in the previous chapters, mastering your physiology, your schedule, and your finances, culminates in this single, powerful state: Presence.

When you have no financial stress, your mind is not wandering to your bills. When you have commanded your time, your mind is not on your next meeting. When your body is fit and rested, you do not feel fatigued. All of this gives you the luxury of being 100% there, in that moment, with that person, with no mental static or internal distractions.

This complete and undivided attention is the rarest and most seductive quality in the modern world. In an age of constant distraction, where everyone is half-listening while scrolling through their phone, offering someone the gift of your full presence communicates, more powerfully than any words, *Right now, in this moment, nothing in the world is more important to me than you.*

This is not a passive state; it is an active skill. It is the foundation upon which all other charismatic tactics are built. Without presence, every other technique is just an empty gesture.

The Presence Switch: Transitioning from Work to Home

Remember the Evening Wind-Down Protocol from Chapter 6? The Presence Switch is its psychological companion.

Many men struggle to transition from work mode to home mode. They carry the stress, the mental checklists, and the unfinished business through the front door. Their partners receive a distracted version of them.

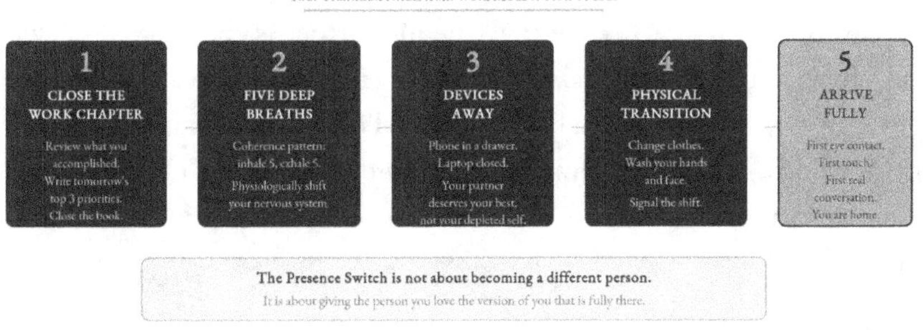

The Presence Switch

The TIS Presence Switch Protocol:

Create a transition ritual. This could be during your commute, or a few minutes in the driveway before entering. The specific activity matters less than the consistency.

Close the work chapter. Mentally review your day and tell yourself: "That chapter is complete. I will return to it tomorrow. Right now, home begins."

Take five deep breaths. This activates your parasympathetic nervous system and signals to your body that the stress response can end.

Set an intention. Before walking through the door, decide: "I will be fully present with my partner tonight."

Leave devices at the door. Literally. Create a charging station near the entrance where phones go when you arrive home.

The Presence Switch is not about becoming a different person. It is about consciously choosing to give your partner the same quality of attention you give to important work. Your partner deserves your best self, not your depleted self.

Tactic 1: The Art of Active Listening (The Power of Silence)

Most people do not listen; they wait for their turn to talk. This is the difference between passive hearing and active listening.

The Lawyer (Passive Hearing): While his partner is speaking, the lawyer is already formulating his rebuttal. He is listening for flaws in her argument, preparing his defense, or waiting for a keyword that allows him to jump in with his own story. He nods, he says "uh-huh," but he is not truly there. His mind is in the future, preparing his next move. The goal is to win the point, not to understand the person.

The Detective (Active Listening): The detective's sole mission is to understand. He completely silences his own internal monologue. His entire focus is on her words, her tone of voice, the emotion behind the words, and what is not being said. He leans in slightly. He holds eye contact. And most critically, he uses the power of the pause, allowing a moment of silence after she finishes speaking to truly absorb what was said before he responds.

To demonstrate this deep level of listening, the detective uses reflective and clarifying language. Instead of "Yeah, I get it," which is dismissive and ends the conversation, try: "So, if I am understanding correctly, it was not the event itself that upset you, but the feeling that you were handling it alone. Is that right?" Or: "It sounds like you felt completely invisible in that meeting. That must have been incredibly frustrating."

This does two powerful things: it confirms that you have accurately received the information, and it makes your partner feel profoundly seen, heard, and valued.

The Bedroom Connection

Active listening does not stop at the bedroom door. In fact, it becomes even more important. A partner who feels unheard during dinner does not suddenly feel heard during intimacy. The patterns of the day carry into the night. But a partner who spent the evening feeling truly listened to carries that emotional connection into physical connection.

Moreover, active listening applies during intimacy itself. Paying attention to her responses, her breathing, her subtle movements, this is listening with your entire body. The same detective mindset that asks *What is she really saying?* also asks *What is her body telling me right now?*

The man who listens well during conversation listens well during intimacy. Both require the same skill: silencing your own agenda and focusing completely on your partner.

Tactic 2: Storytelling (Creating Emotional Connection)

Facts inform, but stories connect. A charismatic man understands that the way to capture a mind and heart is not through a recitation of data, but through a compelling narrative that reveals who he is.

When your partner asks how your day was:

The Factual Answer: "It was busy. Had a lot of meetings, worked on the quarterly report. It was fine." This is a dead end. It provides information but invites no connection.

The Storyteller's Answer: "It was a challenging day. There was a moment this afternoon where we were about to lose that big client, and you could feel the panic rising in the room. But then I shut out all the noise, took a deep breath, and focused on the one single variable we could control. And it worked. It was a good reminder that staying calm under pressure is everything."

The second answer is a story. It has a challenge, a moment of conflict, and a resolution. It reveals your values (calmness under pressure), demonstrates your resilience, and opens a window into your emotional world. This is where your partner connects with the man, not just the professional. Do not be afraid to share small, honest, and vulnerable moments from your own life.

The "Story Spark" Exercise: Think about your day and ask yourself: What was the most frustrating moment? The most satisfying moment? The most surprising moment? The answer to these questions is the spark for a good story.

The Bedroom Connection

Storytelling is foreplay for the mind. Your partner's arousal is deeply connected to emotional engagement. When you share stories that reveal your character, your values, your vulnerabilities, you are creating the emotional intimacy that precedes physical intimacy. The man who shares interesting stories is interesting. The man who reveals his inner world becomes someone his partner wants to know more deeply, in every sense.

Tactic 3: Voice and Tone (The Power of Your Voice)

Research on communication has consistently shown that how you say something matters as much as, and often more than, what you say. While specific percentages vary across studies, the principle is clear: tone, pace, and vocal quality profoundly influence how your message is received.

Your voice is an instrument. Most men never learn to play it.

Pace: Slow Down. Nervous speakers rush. Confident speakers take their time. A slightly slower pace communicates that you are in control, that what you are saying is worth waiting for. Pauses are not awkward silences; they are moments of emphasis. Practice this: Before responding to an important question, pause for a full breath. Let the silence exist. Then answer.

Pitch: Find Your Resonance. A deeper, more resonant voice is generally perceived as more confident. You cannot change your natural voice, but you can learn to speak from your chest rather than your throat. Before important conversations, hum for a few seconds to warm up your vocal cords and find your natural resonance.

Volume: Project Without Shouting. Charismatic speakers project their voice to fill the space without raising volume to the point of aggression. Imagine your voice reaching the person across the room, not just the person in front of you. This creates a sense of command without intimidation.

Variation: Avoid Monotone. A monotone voice, no matter how intelligent the content, puts people to sleep. Vary your pitch, your pace, and your volume to emphasize key points. Let your voice reflect the emotional content of what you are saying.

The Bedroom Connection

Your voice continues to matter during intimacy. The tone you use, the words you whisper, the sounds you make, all communicate desire, reassurance, and connection. A man who has learned to use his voice deliberately can enhance intimate experiences dramatically. Slow, low, deliberate speech creates anticipation. Specific verbal appreciation makes your partner feel desired. Your voice is a tool for connection that does not require physical touch.

Tactic 4: Body Language (The Unspoken Conversation)

Your physical presence communicates powerfully, often more than your words. No matter how powerful your words are, if your body language contradicts them, your body will always win. A man who says, *I am confident,* while slumped over with averted eyes is communicating only one thing: fear.

A charismatic man aligns his words and his body language into a single, congruent message of power and presence.

Posture of Command. Stand and sit up straight. Pull your shoulders back and down, opening up your chest. This does not just signal confidence to others; some research suggests that adopting expansive postures may influence your own psychological state, potentially affecting how confident you feel. How you hold your body affects how you feel.

Calm, Sustained Eye Contact. When your partner is speaking, look into her eyes. Do not stare aggressively, but hold a calm, relaxed gaze. This communicates, "I am focused on you, and every word you say is important." When you speak, it is natural to let your gaze drift occasionally, but always bring it back to connect.

The Power of Non-Sexual Touch: The Oxytocin Bridge. Physical touch, even brief and non-sexual, triggers the release of oxytocin, often called the *bonding hormone*. This hormone creates feelings of trust, connection, and attachment. The bridge to physical intimacy is built with small, non-sexual touches throughout the day. A light touch on her forearm to emphasize a point while talking. A hand on the small of her back as you guide her through a doorway. Holding her hand while laughing at a shared joke. Brushing hair from her face. These small acts build a powerful physical bond, keeping the pilot light of connection lit. They tell your partner, without words, *I am aware of you. I want to be close to you.*

Advanced Tactic: Mirroring. Subtly mirroring your partner's body language is a powerful way to build subconscious rapport. If she leans forward, you lean forward slightly. If she gestures with her right hand, you might later gesture with yours. This should be natural, not a caricature. It sends a signal: "We are in sync."

The Bedroom Connection

Body language does not become irrelevant when you enter the bedroom; it becomes primary. The same principles apply: confident, open posture, sustained eye contact, deliberate, intentional touch. A man who has mastered body language during the day carries that mastery into the night. His touches are confident, not tentative. His gaze is direct, not averted. His body communicates *I want you* before he says a word.

And the oxytocin you have been building all day does not disappear when the lights go out. The non-sexual touches throughout the day have primed both of your bodies for connection. The intimacy you experience at night is the culmi-nation of the intimacy you have been building since morning.

Tactic 5: Building Sexual Tension (The Art of the Slow Burn)

Seduction does not start when you dim the lights. It starts with the morning coffee. A charismatic man knows how to build a slow burn of sexual tension and anticipation throughout the day, so that by the time they are alone, the fire is already roaring.

The Art of the Meaningful Text:

Bad Text: "What do you want for dinner?" (Transactional)

Good Text: "Just thought of you and it made me smile." (Personal and connecting)

TIS-Level Text: "I am still thinking about the way you laughed last night. Cannot wait to see you tonight." (Specific, complimentary, and builds anticipation)

The Power of the Specific Compliment:

Generic Compliment: "You look beautiful." (Nice, but generic. She has heard it before.)

Specific Compliment: "The way your eyes lit up when you were talking about your project today was incredible. Your passion is so attractive." (This compliments her essence, not just her appearance, and shows you were actively listening.)

Future Pacing: Planting Seeds of Anticipation. Future pacing is the art of planting a seed of a future event in her mind. "I have been thinking about what we are going to do this weekend..." or "I cannot wait for our connection night on Thursday" creates a shared sense of anticipation and excitement. It makes her an active participant in the seduction. "I am planning something special for us. You will have to wait to find out." "There is something I have been wanting to try with you..."

All three men discovered that the slow burn changed everything.

John, the introvert, found his version in meaningful texts. "I used to send her logistics," he admitted. "'What time are you home?' 'Should I pick up milk?' Now I send her one real message a day. Something specific I noticed about her. Something I'm looking forward to. She told me she reads them multiple times."

Matt implemented future pacing. "I started telling her what I was planning for our connection nights. Not everything, just enough to build anticipation. She said she thinks about it all day now. That she's already in the mood before I get home."

David focused on specific compliments. "I used to say 'you look nice.' Now I say exactly what I noticed and why it affected me. Her eyes. Her laugh. The way she handled something with the kids. She told me she feels seen for the first time in years."

The slow burn is not a technique separate from intimacy. It is where intimacy begins. Charisma is not the art of manipulation. It is the art of creating an authentic connection by translating your internal strength and your sincere interest into words and actions that make your partner feel seen, desired, and safe. When you build this connection, the bedroom becomes the natural and passionate celebration of that deep bond.

For the Charisma Micro-Challenges, Conversation Starters, and the complete Connection Toolkit, see Appendix F.

Commander's Q&A: Charisma Operations

I am an introvert. This all sounds exhausting and unnatural for me.

This is a critical misunderstanding of charisma. Charisma is not about being the loudest person in the room. Some of the most charismatic people are quiet and reserved. Charisma is about the quality of your attention, not the quantity of your words. Active listening, sustained eye contact, and being fully present are actually introvert superpowers. They do not drain your energy; they focus it. You do not have to be the life of the party; you just have to be the most present person in the conversation.

Is this not just a form of manipulation or "playing a game"?

The line between charisma and manipulation is defined by one thing: intent. Manipulation is using these techniques to get something from someone for your own selfish benefit. Charisma is using these techniques to make someone feel seen, valued, and desired, for the mutual benefit of strengthening your connection. If your intent is to genuinely understand and connect with your partner, these tactics are simply the tools to express that intent effectively. A hammer can build a house or break a window. The tool is neutral; the intent defines the outcome.

What if I try this and it feels awkward or I mess up?

You will. Learning any new skill feels awkward at first. The key is to have a sense of humor about it. You can even say to your partner, "I am practicing being a better listener, so if I seem intensely focused, that is why!" Being open about your intent turns awkwardness into a shared, charming experience. It also invites your partner to support your growth rather than be confused by sudden behavioral changes.

My partner does not seem receptive to compliments or texts. What should I do?

First, consider whether you have built up enough "presence credit" through consistent listening and attention. Compliments without the foundation of genuine presence can feel hollow or transactional. Second, pay attention to how your partner receives appreciation. Some people respond better to words, others to touch, others to acts of service. If verbal compliments do not resonate, try non-verbal appreciation: sustained eye contact, physical touch, doing something thoughtful. Third, be patient. If your partner is not accustomed to this kind of attention from you, they may initially be skeptical. Consistency over time builds trust.

Commander's Briefing: Chapter 8

- **Charisma is Not a Gift; It is a Tactic.** Your internal power is useless without a bridge to the external world. Charisma is that bridge. Great sex begins long before the bedroom, ignited by the connection you build all day long.

- **The Foundation is Presence.** Undivided attention is the rarest and most seductive quality in the modern world. It communicates, "In this moment, nothing is more important than you."

- **Use the Presence Switch.** Create a deliberate ritual to transition from work mode to home mode. Close the work chapter with five deep breaths and a conscious intention. Leave devices at the door. Your partner deserves your best self, not your depleted self.

- **Listen Like a Detective, Not a Lawyer.** Most people wait for their turn to talk. A commander listens to understand. Silence your internal monologue, absorb their words, and use reflective language to show you have truly heard them.

- **Facts Inform; Stories Connect.** Do not just report your day; tell its story. A narrative with a challenge and a resolution reveals your character and values, opening a window for true connection. Storytelling is foreplay for the mind.

- **Master Your Voice.** Pace, pitch, volume, and variation all communicate confidence and presence. Your voice is an instrument. Slow down. Find your resonance. Let silence work for you.

- **Your Body Language is the Unspoken Conversation.** Align your physical presence with your words. Command your posture, maintain calm and sustained eye contact, and use small, non-sexual touches to build a constant current of oxytocin and connection throughout the day.

- **Seduction is a Slow Burn, Not a Switch.** Build sexual tension throughout the day with meaningful texts, specific compliments, and the art of future pacing. By the time you are alone together, the fire should already be roaring.

- **Three Versions, One Lesson.** Charisma failures follow three patterns: the introvert myth (believing presence requires extroversion, when attention quality is the true currency), the presence leak (giving your best energy to work and your depleted remainder to home), and selective deployment (treating charisma as a limited professional resource rather than a muscle that strengthens with use at home). Identify your pattern and redirect your energy where it matters most.

Chapter 9

The Advanced Arsenal: From Control to Artistry

Beyond the Basics

The texts started arriving within weeks of each other.

John: "Something shifted. I don't think about control anymore. I just... have it. What's next?"

Matt: "Thirty minutes used to feel like a race against the clock. Now it feels like I could go indefinitely. Is this normal?"

David: "We did it. Synchronized. On purpose. She cried afterward. Good tears. What else is possible?"

Three men who had started as anxious beginners were now asking the question that separates competence from mastery: What else is possible?

I had been waiting for this question. Because the techniques I had taught them so far, *The Reset*, *The Breath*, *The Rhythm*, were foundations, not ceilings. They were the scales a pianist practices before attempting a concerto.

Any competent driver can get a car from Point A to Point B safely. He can obey the traffic laws, stay in his lane, and arrive at his destination. But a Formula 1 pilot is a different species. A racing pilot does not just drive the car; he pushes it to its absolute limits. He understands every nuance of the engine, every degree of grip in the tires, and every curve of the track. He does not just complete the journey;

he crafts every moment of it into a symphony of speed, control, and precision. He does not follow the map; he becomes the master of the terrain itself.

You have built the foundation. The Reset gives you control over your ejaculatory reflex. The Breath keeps your nervous system calm. The Rhythm creates the wave patterns that synchronize your arousal with your partner's. But control is not the destination. Control is the vehicle. The destination is mastery: the ability to not merely last, but to shape the experience. To read your partner's responses in real time and adjust. To build pleasure deliberately, like a composer arranging a symphony. To transform what was once an anxious performance into a collaborative art form.

At this level, you stop thinking about avoiding failure and start thinking about creating excellence. A man focused on not finishing too soon is defensive, reactive, trapped in his own head. A man focused on crafting an unforgettable experience is expansive, creative, completely present with his partner.

The Reset, The Breath, and The Rhythm are not techniques you master once and forget. They are powers that strengthen with practice, that become faster and more automatic with each use. The more you train your pelvic floor, the quicker you can complete a Reset. The more you practice coherence breathing, the faster you return to calm. The more familiar you become with The Rhythm, the more naturally it flows.

This is not a pass-fail examination. It is a journey of continuous improvement. If your Reset currently takes twenty seconds, with practice it may take fifteen, then twelve. If you currently need to withdraw to execute a Reset, with practice you may be able to do it while remaining inside your partner. If you currently need to consciously count your breaths, with practice the pattern becomes automatic. Every session is training. Every intimate encounter builds your capacity. And if you experience setbacks, if the reflex catches you off guard, remember: this is not failure. It is feedback. It is data that tells you where to focus your practice next.

John, Matt, and David each reached this level at different speeds. John's engineering mindset made him a natural at systematic practice; he progressed fastest. Matt's unpredictable schedule meant his practice was inconsistent, but his intensity during available windows compensated. David's fifteen years of partnership with his wife meant he had the deepest communication foundation to build on.

Your journey will have its own pace. What matters is not how quickly you progress, but that you continue progressing. This chapter gives you the advanced tactics that become available as your foundation strengthens.

Three Men, Three Mastery Journeys

John's Advanced Reset Journey

John's question came over the fence on a Saturday morning.

"I want to try The Reset while I'm inside her," he said, keeping his voice low. "I've been practicing solo and it works perfectly. But I'm nervous about trying it for real."

"What's the fear?"

"That it won't work. That I'll lose control anyway. That she'll feel like she's part of some... experiment."

"Have you talked to her about it?"

He shook his head.

"That's where you start," I said. "Not with technique. With communication. Tell her what you've been practicing. Tell her what you want to try. Make her your partner in this, not a test subject."

A week later, he texted me: "It worked. Three times. She said it was the sexiest thing she's ever experienced."

John had been practicing The Reset for several weeks.

Solo sessions had taught him to recognize the edge, to contract his pelvic floor at maximum intensity the moment he felt the ejaculatory reflex approaching, and to hold that contraction while focusing on his breath cycles rather than counting seconds.

He had learned that one and a half breath cycles, a slow inhale for five counts, a slow exhale for five counts, and another slow inhale, gave him approximately fifteen seconds of hold time. Two full cycles brought him to twenty seconds.

By focusing on breath cycles rather than watching the clock, he stayed present with his body rather than anxious about time.

After three successful solo sessions where he executed multiple Resets without losing his erection, John felt ready to try it with his girlfriend.

"I want to try something tonight," he told her before they began. "I have been practicing a technique that gives me more control. Tonight, I want to try it while I am inside you."

She was intrigued. "What do I need to do?"

"When I say 'hold,' I need you to stay as still as possible. Keep kissing me, touch my face, my chest, stay connected with me. But minimize any movement that stimulates my penis. I will be doing an internal contraction and focusing on my breathing. It takes about fifteen to twenty seconds. Then I will say 'go' and we continue."

The first time he called "hold," she felt him tense inside her. She could sense his intense focus, his deliberate breathing. She kissed his neck softly, ran her fingers through his hair, whispered "I am right here" against his ear. Fifteen seconds passed. Twenty.

"Go," he breathed, and they resumed.

They did this three times that night. Each time, John felt more confident. The Reset worked inside her just as it worked during solo practice. His erection remained strong throughout.

And something unexpected happened: his girlfriend found the pauses intensely erotic.

"There is something incredibly sexy about feeling you fight for control," she told him afterward. "Feeling you hold back, knowing you want me so much that you have to actively resist. It made me feel... powerful. Desired."

John had discovered that The Reset was not an interruption of intimacy. It was an intensification of it.

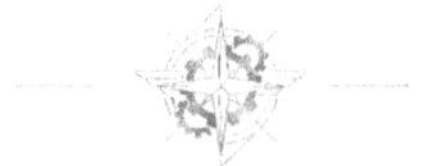

Matt's Integrated System Mastery

Matt's breakthrough came from an unexpected realization.

"I've been treating this like three separate systems," he told me during a school pickup. "The Reset. The Breath. The Rhythm. Three things to manage. Three things to think about. It's exhausting."

"And?"

"What if they're not three things? What if they're one thing that I've been artificially separating?"

I smiled. This was the insight I had been waiting for him to reach on his own.

"Your body already knows how to integrate them," I said. "You've been practicing each piece. Now stop practicing the pieces and let them merge. Trust that your training has prepared your body to respond automatically. Your job isn't to manage the system anymore. Your job is to be present with your wife while the system manages itself."

The shift happened gradually. His pelvic floor, strengthened by weeks of daily training, now responded automatically to rising arousal. He did not need to think *contract now*; his body recognized the warning signs and initiated The Reset instinctively. His breathing had become a background rhythm, steady and calm without conscious attention. The Rhythm had become intuitive, his body naturally varying depth and pace based on his arousal level and her responses.

"Now," he told his wife, "thirty minutes feels completely different. I am not racing against the clock or fighting my body. I am in command of the experience. I can speed up when you want intensity. I can slow down when I need to recalibrate.

I can extend or contract the experience based on what we both need in that moment."

His wife noticed the transformation. "You used to feel… desperate," she said carefully. "Like you were trying to accomplish something before time ran out. Now you feel… present. Confident. Like however long we have is exactly right."

Matt had learned that mastery was not about duration. It was about command.

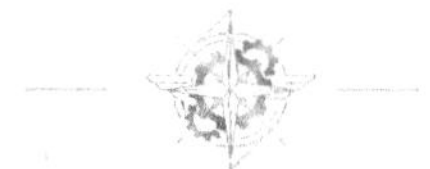

David's Synchronized Crescendo

David called me with a question I had never heard from him before.

"Is it actually possible to… time it? Both of us finishing at the same moment? On purpose?"

"Yes."

Silence. Then: "We've been together fifteen years. It's happened maybe twice. By accident. Are you telling me we could do it deliberately?"

"With practice. With communication. With your Reset skills."

I explained the plateau technique: holding yourself at an eight or nine while communicating with your partner about her arousal level.

Building her while maintaining yourself. Timing the final ascent together.

"It sounds complicated," he said.

"It requires practice. But you have the foundation. Your Reset is strong enough to hold a plateau. The question is whether you and your wife can communicate that openly during intimacy."

"We've never talked that directly during… you know."

"Then that's where you start. Not with the technique. With the conversation about the technique."

Two weeks later, he called me. His voice was different. Quieter. Almost reverent.

"We did it," he said. "First try didn't work. Second try was close. Third try..."

He paused.

"She cried. I almost did too. It was like... I don't know how to describe it. Like we were the same person for a moment."

Using the communication techniques from Chapter 4, they had developed a simple system.

During intimate moments, she would tell him where she was on a one-to-ten scale. He would use The Reset to hold himself at a high plateau, around eight or nine, while continuing to focus on her pleasure.

"I am at seven," she would whisper.

Then, minutes later, "Eight. Getting close."

He would adjust his rhythm, building her arousal while executing micro-Resets to maintain his own controlled plateau. When she said "nine," he would begin his own final ascent, timing his release to coincide with hers.

The first time they achieved it deliberately, his wife was overwhelmed.

Not just from the physical intensity, though that was unlike anything they had experienced together. From the profound intimacy of choosing to cross that threshold as one.

"It felt like we were completely synchronized," she said, tears in her eyes. "I have never felt so... cherished. So prioritized."

When both partners experience this level of connection, the bond deepens in ways that extend far beyond the bedroom.

This is the hidden reward of mastery: not just better technique, but deeper connection.

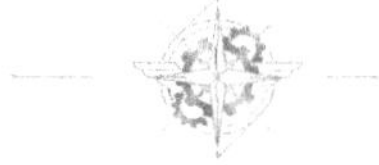

A Note on Consent and Communication

Before we proceed to the advanced tactics, a critical reminder.

These techniques involve deliberate management of arousal, yours and your partner's. They require a level of communication and mutual enthusiasm that goes beyond basic intimacy. Your partner must be an informed, willing participant, not a passive recipient of techniques she does not understand.

Before attempting any advanced tactic:

Discuss it outside the bedroom. Explain what you want to try and why. Use the communication frameworks from Chapter 4. Invite questions. Address concerns.

Establish clear signals. During advanced play, both partners need ways to communicate comfort levels. A simple "green light / yellow light / red light" system works well. Green means continue. Yellow means slow down or check in. Red means stop immediately.

Debrief afterward. What worked? What did not? What would each of you like to try differently next time? This feedback loop is essential for mutual growth.

Respect boundaries absolutely. If your partner is not enthusiastic about a particular technique, do not push. Advanced tactics only enhance intimacy when both partners are fully engaged. Reluctant participation undermines everything.

The goal of the Advanced Arsenal is not to demonstrate your prowess. It is to create experiences of profound connection. That connection requires trust, communication, and mutual enthusiasm. Without these, technique is meaningless.

Advanced Tactic 1: The Reset Amplification (Harnessing the Edging Effect)

You may have heard of *edging*, the practice of approaching orgasm and then pulling back, repeatedly, to intensify the eventual release. The concept has existed for centuries. But traditional edging has significant limitations: it often requires complete withdrawal, it depends on uncertain timing, and it frequently results in lost erections or accidental climaxes.

The Reset transforms edging from an uncertain art into a precise science.

With The Reset, you are not simply "pulling back" and hoping the arousal subsides. You are actively commanding your ejaculatory reflex to stand down. You are using the physiological principle of muscle fatigue to create a reliable window of control. And critically, you can do this without withdrawing, without losing your erection, and with predictable results.

When you use The Reset at the edge of climax, three things happen:

Accumulated Arousal. Research suggests that repeatedly approaching and retreating from the edge may enhance the eventual release, as the body builds arousal without the neurochemical reset that follows orgasm. By executing The Reset at the edge, you prevent the release of prolactin (the *satisfaction* hormone that induces the refractory period after orgasm) from entering your system. This allows arousal to accumulate to levels you have never experienced before.

Heightened Sensitivity. Many men report that each cycle of approaching the edge and executing a Reset increases the overall intensity of sensation. The pleasure you feel at intensity level seven after three Reset cycles is far more powerful than the pleasure you felt at level seven before you started. You are not just delaying release; you are amplifying the capacity for pleasure itself.

Maintained Control. Unlike traditional edging, which depends on guessing when to stop, The Reset gives you a mechanical intervention that works regardless of timing. Even if you misjudge and begin the ejaculatory reflex, a strong Reset contraction may significantly delay it. And unlike traditional edging, which often requires complete cessation of stimulation, The Reset allows you to remain inside your partner, maintaining connection and her arousal while you regain control.

When you finally choose to cross the threshold, the resulting orgasm is significantly more intense. It is not a localized event; it is a systemic release that can feel like it courses through your entire body. Multiple Reset cycles at the edge create an orgasm that is qualitatively different from anything you have experienced before.

The critical difference from traditional edging: The Reset takes twelve to twenty seconds, not minutes. It works with reliability, not hope. And it preserves your erection throughout. You get the amplification benefits of edging with the precision of the TIS system.

Three Levels of Reset Amplification

Level 1: Solo Calibration

Before attempting Reset Amplification with a partner, master the technique in solo practice.

Step 1: Establish Your Baseline. Begin a solo session with coherence breathing already active. Slow inhale for a count of five, slow exhale for a count of five. This calm state is your starting point.

Step 2: Build Toward the Edge. Slowly increase your arousal. Your mission is to recognize, with absolute clarity, the very beginning of the ejaculatory reflex. This is not the point of no return; this is the warning signal that precedes it. Pay exquisite attention to this sensation. Learn to recognize it earlier and earlier.

Step 3: Execute The Reset at the Edge. The moment you feel the warning signs, contract your pelvic floor at maximum intensity. Do not count seconds; instead, focus on your breath cycles. One complete cycle (inhale for five, exhale for five) is approximately ten seconds. One and a half cycles brings you to fifteen seconds. Two full cycles is twenty seconds. Hold the contraction while breathing. Feel the ejaculatory pressure retreat. Many men describe it as the sensation *dropping back* or *draining away.*

Step 4: Resume and Repeat. Once the contraction releases and the reflex has retreated, resume stimulation. Build toward the edge again. Execute another Reset. In a single session, practice two to three Reset cycles before allowing yourself to finish. Notice how the eventual orgasm differs from your normal experience. This is the amplification effect in action.

Level 2: Partner Integration (Inside Reset)

This is where The Reset becomes truly powerful: executing it while remaining inside your partner.

The Setup: Explain to your partner what you are practicing. You might say: "I want to try holding The Reset while I am inside you. When I say 'hold,' I need you to stay as still as possible. Keep kissing me, touching my face and chest, stay connected with me, but minimize any movement that stimulates my penis. I will be doing an internal contraction and focusing on my breathing. It takes about fifteen to twenty seconds, maybe one and a half to two breath cycles. Then I will say 'continue' and we resume."

The Execution: When you feel the warning signs of approaching climax, say your cue word. Your partner stills. You execute The Reset: maximum pelvic floor contraction while maintaining your coherence breathing. Focus on completing one and a half to two breath cycles rather than counting seconds. Feel the reflex retreat. Feel your control return. Say your continuation cue. Resume.

The Benefits: Your erection remains strong because you never withdrew. Your partner stays aroused because connection was maintained. The pause becomes part of the experience, not an interruption. Her awareness of your controlled struggle often heightens her arousal.

The Learning Curve: Your first attempts may not succeed perfectly. The stimulation of remaining inside your partner makes The Reset more challenging than in solo practice. This is normal. Start with Inside Resets when your arousal is at level six or seven, not level nine. As your pelvic floor strengthens and your technique improves, you will be able to execute Inside Resets at higher arousal levels.

Level 3: The Flow State (Micro-Reset Integration)

At this level, The Reset becomes so integrated with your movement that you no longer need to stop. You execute *micro-Resets* continuously, riding the edge indefinitely.

The Technique: As you approach higher arousal levels, you begin incorporating brief pelvic floor contractions into your rhythm. These are not full twenty-second Resets; they are five to ten second pulses that prevent arousal from tipping over the edge. Simultaneously, you shift to predominantly shallow movements. The reduced stimulation, combined with the micro-Reset contractions, allows you to maintain a high plateau of arousal without crossing the threshold.

The Breath-Reset-Rhythm Integration: This is where all three tactics merge into a single flowing system. Your coherence breathing continues automatically, keeping your nervous system calm. Your pelvic floor pulses with brief contractions, managing your arousal level. Your rhythm shifts between shallow and deep, varying stimulation intensity. You are no longer thinking about three separate techniques. You are experiencing one integrated state of controlled pleasure. Your body manages itself while your mind remains free to focus entirely on your partner, her responses, her pleasure, her experience.

This is the level of attentiveness that transforms how your partner experiences you. Not because of physical attributes or techniques, but because of what you make her feel: prioritized, present, completely focused on the shared experience. When both partners feel truly prioritized, truly satisfied, the bond deepens in ways that extend far beyond the bedroom. This is the hidden reward of mastery: not just better technique, but deeper connection.

Advanced Tactic 2: Orgasmic Variety (Exploring Your Partner's Map)

Mastery is not just about controlling your own experience; it is about conducting your partner's experience like a virtuoso.

The female orgasm is not a single, monolithic event. It is a vast and varied landscape, with different peaks that are reached by different paths. A beginner is happy to find one path and stick to it. A master knows the entire map and enjoys exploring every trail.

Now that you have the gift of time and presence, you have the luxury of exploring this landscape with her.

Think of yourself as a music producer in a recording studio. A novice just turns up the volume on all the instruments at once. The master knows that the magic is in the mix. He knows when to feature the bass line (deep, resonant stimulation), when to bring in the high notes (light, teasing touch), and when to combine them for a powerful crescendo.

Becoming a Master Mixer

Map the Terrain. The only way to learn the map is to ask the local guide. Open, curious, non-judgmental communication is essential. Instead of "Did you come?" (a pass/fail question that creates pressure), try: "Tell me what that felt like. Was it more of a deep, warm feeling, or a sharp, electric one?" Use a scale for real-time feedback: "Where are you on the arousal scale right now?" This gives you invaluable data to work with, allowing you to adjust in the moment.

Master the Instruments. Clitoral stimulation: Understand that for the vast majority of women, this is the primary pathway to orgasm. It is one of the most densely innervated areas of the body. Learn to integrate consistent, rhythmic manual or oral stimulation even during intercourse. This is not *foreplay*; this is part of the main event. Experiment with different types of touch: light circles, direct pressure, tapping, vibration. Listen to her feedback. What works varies significantly between individuals and even between encounters.

Internal stimulation often produces a deeper, more full-bodied sensation. Experiment with positions and angles that allow for varied depths and pressures. A simple adjustment in angle or rhythm can make a significant difference.

Blended experiences represent the peak of the art form. This is when you combine multiple forms of stimulation simultaneously, creating layers of sensation that build on each other. This is the full orchestra playing in perfect harmony.

Synchronized Climax: The Ultimate Shared Experience

With The Reset mastery you have developed, simultaneous climax is no longer a matter of luck but a plannable achievement. By using The Reset to hold yourself at a high plateau (around eight or nine) and actively communicating with your partner to bring her to her own peak, you can make the conscious decision to cross the finish line together.

This requires your mastery of The Reset to maintain your plateau, her willingness to communicate her arousal level, and mutual trust and practice. The first few attempts may miss the mark. That is fine. The practice itself is pleasurable. And when you finally achieve it, the experience of sharing that moment of release is profoundly connecting.

Advanced Tactic 3: The Strategic Use of Positions

Beginners change positions for random variety or because they saw something in a movie. Masters change them for tactical advantage. Each position offers a different level of control for you, a different depth, and a different focus of stimulation for her.

STRATEGIC POSITION USE

Fluid Transitions Between Control and Intensity

CONTROL-FOCUSED	INTENSITY-FOCUSED
The Command Center: Your Safe Harbor	The Advance: When Control is Confident
When to use:	**When to use:**
Practicing Inside Resets	Control is established and confident
Recalibrating after arousal spike	Building toward shared climax
Building confidence with technique	Maximizing mutual pleasure
Characteristics:	**Characteristics:**
You control depth, pace, and rhythm	Higher stimulation, deeper connection

Transitions should feel like dance moves, not furniture rearrangement.
Consent and communication are non-negotiable. Discuss preferences outside the bedroom.

Control-Focused Positions (The Command Center)

Positions where you are less physically active and can easily control the depth and pace are your training ground and your *Safe Harbor*. Examples include partner on top where she controls the rhythm, side-lying positions, and seated positions with her on your lap facing you. These are perfect for practicing Inside Resets or for moments when you need to lower your arousal level. If you feel yourself getting too close to the edge in a more intense position, a smooth transition to one of these can be your tactical pivot.

Intensity-Focused Positions (The Advance).
When you are completely confident in your control and want to maximize intensity for both of you. Positions that allow deeper angles, standing positions, and positions that allow simultaneous manual stimulation. These allow for deeper stimulation and more powerful movement. Transitioning fluidly from a control position to an intensity position and back again is the mark of a confident commander who is a master of pacing.

The Fluid Transition.
The art is in the seamless movement between positions. A clumsy position change breaks the flow and can feel mechanical. A smooth transition feels like a natural evolution of the experience. Practice transitions during lower-stakes moments so they become second nature. The goal is for position changes to feel like dance moves, not furniture rearrangement.

For foundational Reset training, see Appendix E: Pelvic Floor Training Fundamentals.

For advanced digital training tools with personalized guidance, visit tismethod. com/tactical-intimacy/book-owners

Commander's Q&A: Advanced Operations

I executed The Reset successfully, but a few seconds later the ejaculatory reflex returned immediately. What went wrong?

Nothing went wrong. This is normal, especially in highly arousing situations. Having just completed a Reset does not prevent you from needing another one immediately if stimulation or excitement spikes suddenly. Your pelvic floor recovered some contractile strength during those few seconds. If the reflex returns, execute another Reset immediately. You can do multiple Resets in quick succession if needed. There is no "cooldown period" required. With practice, you will learn to read the post-Reset period better. You will learn how much stimulation you can handle immediately after a Reset versus how much requires you to ease back in gradually. This calibration comes through experience.

I am worried that The Reset will not work in high-arousal situations with my partner. It seems easier in solo practice.

You are correct that partner situations are more challenging. The stimulation is different, the emotional intensity is higher, and there are elements you cannot control. Start with Inside Resets at lower arousal levels (six or seven) rather than waiting until you are at the edge (nine). As your technique strengthens, gradually attempt Resets at higher arousal levels. Build your confidence progressively. Also remember: even if a Reset does not completely halt the reflex, it often delays it significantly. A partial success is still success. You are building skill with each attempt.

Will my partner not think this is all just a game or a performance?

This comes back to your intent and your communication. If your intent is to demonstrate endurance for your own ego, it will feel like a performance. If your intent, which you communicate clearly, is "I have developed this control so I can focus completely on your pleasure," it becomes a gift. Frame it as something you are doing for the relationship, not something you are doing to impress.

This seems like a lot to think about. How do I stay present?

This is the paradox of mastery. To achieve a state of effortless presence, you must first go through a period of intense, conscious practice. A concert pianist is not thinking about where his fingers go during a performance; he has practiced the scales so many thousands of times that his fingers move on their own, freeing his mind to focus on the music and emotion. The three TIS tactics are your scales. Practice them, and they will become second nature. The goal is unconscious competence: mastery so complete that it requires no thought, leaving your full attention available for your partner.

My partner seems uncomfortable with the communication required for synchronized climax. How do I proceed?

Do not push. Some partners are not comfortable with explicit verbal communication during intimacy, and that is perfectly valid. You can gather information through non-verbal cues: her breathing, her movements, her sounds. Over time, you will learn to read these signals accurately. Synchronized climax becomes possible through attunement rather than explicit communication. Alternatively, start smaller. Instead of asking for a numerical scale, simply ask her to squeeze your hand when she is getting close. This requires less verbal articulation and may feel more natural. The goal is connection, not compliance with a specific technique.

Commander's Briefing: Chapter 9

- **Transition from Competence to Artistry.** You are no longer just driving the car; you are becoming a racing pilot. Control is the vehicle; mastery is the destination. Stop thinking about avoiding failure and start thinking about creating excellence.

- **Your Foundation Strengthens With Practice.** The Reset, The Breath, and The Rhythm become faster, more automatic, and more powerful with continued use. Every session is training. Setbacks are not failure; they are feedback.

- **Consent and Communication are Non-Negotiable.** Advanced tactics require informed, enthusiastic participation from your partner. Discuss techniques outside the bedroom. Establish clear signals (green/yellow/red). Debrief afterward. Respect boundaries absolutely.

- **Advanced Tactic 1: Reset Amplification.** Unlike uncertain traditional edging, The Reset gives you precise control at the edge of climax. Research suggests that repeatedly approaching and retreating from the edge may enhance the eventual release. Three levels of mastery: Solo Calibration (breath-cycle-based holds), Inside Reset with partner (maintaining connection while executing), and Flow State integration (micro-Resets woven into continuous rhythm).

- **Advanced Tactic 2: Exploring Your Partner's Map.** Mastery extends beyond your own control to conducting her experience. With the gift of time, explore the full landscape of her pleasure. Map the terrain through curious communication. Master the instruments: clitoral, internal, and blended stimulation. Build toward synchronized climax using plateau control and real-time communication.

- **Advanced Tactic 3: Strategic Position Use.** Control-focused positions are your Safe Harbor for practicing Inside Resets and recalibrating. Intensity-focused positions are your advance when control is confident. Fluid transitions between them mark true mastery; position changes should feel like dance moves, not furniture rearrangement.

- **The Hidden Reward of Mastery.** When both partners feel truly prioritized and satisfied, the bond deepens far beyond the bedroom. This is not just better technique; it is deeper connection.

- **Three Mastery Paths.** Advanced mastery develops along three dimensions: precision (executing Inside Resets with a partner while maintaining connection), integration (merging three separate techniques into one automatic system), and synchronization (using plateau control and real-time communication to share the climactic moment). Each dimension builds on your growing foundation.

CHAPTER 10

THE LEGACY TACTIC: FROM BEDROOM MASTERY TO LIFE MASTERY

The Question That Changed Everything

THE QUESTION CAME FROM Matt, but it could have come from any of them.

We were at a school event, watching our kids perform in a holiday concert. Matt leaned over during a pause between songs.

"I've been thinking," he said quietly. "I've mastered the techniques. I can last as long as I want. But yesterday I snapped at my son over spilled milk. The same man who held a beating heart steady that morning couldn't hold his patience for five seconds at home."

He paused, watching his son on stage.

"What's the point of control in the bedroom if I can't control myself everywhere else?"

It was the question I had been waiting for. The question that meant he was ready for the final lesson.

John had arrived at it differently. "I'm present with her during intimacy," he told me. "Completely focused. But the moment we're done, I reach for my phone. She said I'm 'here but not here.' She's right."

David's version cut deepest. At 41, with fifteen years of marriage behind him, he was thinking about what would endure long after the projects were finished and the paychecks spent. "What will they remember about me?" he asked one evening. "My family. When I'm gone. I want them to remember a man who was present. Who listened. Who stayed calm when things got hard. But I'm not sure that's what they're experiencing right now."

Three men who had mastered the bedroom. Three men who sensed that mastery had a larger purpose.

What is a man's legacy? Is it the number in his bank account? The title on his business card? These are achievements, and they are worthy of respect. But they are not a legacy. Achievements are etched in stone, monuments to what a man did. A legacy is written in the hearts of others, a testament to who a man was. It is the warmth people feel when they speak your name. It is the stories they tell about how you made them feel, the strength you gave them, the safety you provided.

You began this book on a journey. Perhaps you came here hoping to fix a "problem," a frustrating mechanical issue that felt disconnected from the rest of your successful life. But as you progressed through these pages, you discovered that the *Tactical Intimacy System* is not just a set of techniques for the bedroom; it is a complete operating system for a life of command, presence, and connection.

The quality of your intimate life is inseparable from the quality of your entire relationship. You can master every technique in this book. But if you walk out of the bedroom and become distracted, dismissive, or reactive, those bedroom victories become isolated events rather than expressions of a deeper connection. This chapter is about completing the circuit. It is about taking the powers you have developed and applying them to become not just a masterful lover, but a legendary partner, a present father, and a man whose legacy will be written in the hearts of those he loves.

Three Men, Three Legacy Journeys

I gave each of them the same challenge.

"You've mastered control in the most intense, vulnerable environment imaginable," I said. "Now take that same discipline, the breathing, the presence, the self-regulation, and apply it to every other room in your house. Every other moment in your life."

John looked skeptical. "It's not the same thing."

"It's exactly the same thing," I said. "The muscle you built to control your ejaculatory reflex is the same muscle that controls your temper. The presence you cultivated to read your partner's responses is the same presence that makes your family feel truly seen. You've been training for this without realizing it."

Matt nodded slowly. "The bedroom was the dojo."

"And the world is your stage," I finished. "Let me show you how to step onto it."

John's Presence Transformation

John's girlfriend had said the words so many times that they had lost their impact. But when he repeated them to me over the fence, I heard something different in his voice.

"She says I'm 'here but not here.' And she's right.

I can be completely present with her during intimacy, focused, attentive, reading every response. But the moment we leave the bedroom, that presence evaporates."

"Where does it go?" I asked.

He held up his phone. "Here. Always here. Or thinking about code. Or planning tomorrow. I give her my full attention for thirty minutes in the bedroom and my divided attention for the other twenty-three hours."

"So you already know how to be present. You just don't do it consistently."

He was quiet for a moment. "I never thought of it that way."

"The Daily Presence Drill," I said.

"Ten minutes. Every evening. No phone. No laptop. Just her. Treat it with the same seriousness you treat your TIS practice."

"Ten minutes doesn't sound like much."

"It's not about duration. It's about consistency. Ten minutes of real presence, every single day, will transform your relationship more than occasional hours of half-attention."

The first few nights felt awkward.

He kept reaching for his phone out of habit. His mind wandered to work problems. But he persisted, using the same *coherence breathing* that helped him maintain calm during intimacy to quiet his restless thoughts.

By the third week, something shifted. He started noticing things he had missed before. The way her eyes lit up when she talked about her sister. The subtle tension in her shoulders when work stressed her. The specific laugh she saved for his terrible jokes.

"You see me now," she said one evening, her voice soft with emotion. "Like, really see me."

John realized that the presence he had learned in the bedroom had trained him for something far more valuable: the ability to be fully present with the person he loved. And that presence, extended into every interaction, had transformed their relationship more profoundly than any bedroom technique ever could.

"The strange thing," he told her, "is that our intimate life has gotten even better. Not because I am doing anything different in those moments, but because of everything I am doing differently in all the other moments."

She smiled. "I feel closer to you now. All the time. That makes me want you more."

Presence in life fed desire in the bedroom. Mastery in the bedroom fed presence in life. The connection was seamless.

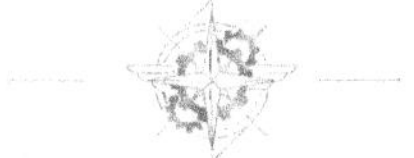

Matt's Calm Captain

Matt had always been two different people. At the hospital, he was unshakeable. His team called him "The Immune" because nothing seemed to penetrate his composure. When the emergency room erupted into chaos, Matt became calmer, more focused, more present.

At home, with his son and daughter, he was something else entirely. Short-tempered. Distant. The stress he managed so masterfully at work seemed to explode the moment he walked through the front door.

His eight-year-old son said something that changed everything.

Matt had snapped at him for leaving toys on the stairs. It was not a big explosion, just the irritated, impatient tone that had become his default at home. He had immediately followed it with "I love you, buddy" as he always did, trying to soften the edge.

His son looked up at him, confused and hurt. "Dad, is this what love means?"

The question hit Matt like a physical blow. His son was genuinely asking. He had heard "I love you" so many times, but what he had experienced was impatience, distraction, and irritation. In his eight-year-old mind, he was trying to reconcile the words with the reality.

That night, Matt made a decision. He would become "The Immune" at home, not by suppressing his emotions, but by regulating them.

He started implementing the same techniques at home that he used in the operating room and in the bedroom. The *Presence Switch* before walking through the door, consciously leaving work stress in the car. Coherence breathing when his daughter's whining threatened to trigger frustration. Conscious pauses, a slow breath for a count of five, before responding to his son's endless questions.

The transformation was not instant, but it was steady. His wife noticed first. "You are calmer," she observed one evening. "Even when everything is chaos, you are steady. What changed?"

"I realized I was giving everyone else the captain," Matt said. "And giving you the exhausted crew member. You deserve the captain too."

His son noticed next. One evening, he approached Matt hesitantly. "Daddy, can we play Legos?"

In the past, Matt might have said "in a minute" while continuing to scroll his phone. This time, he put down his phone immediately. "Absolutely. Show me what you are building."

For the next thirty minutes, he was fully present. No phone. No mental review of cases. Just his son, the Legos, and the simple joy of building something together.

When they finished, his son hugged him. "This is what love means," he said quietly.

Matt held him tight, tears in his eyes. He was finally the same man at home that he was at work: the calm captain his family needed. And the man his wife desired.

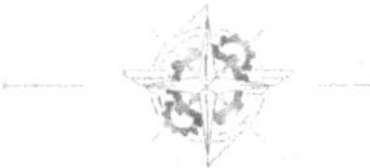

David's Legacy Perspective

David's question came from a deeper place than technique or skill.

"What will they remember?" he asked me one evening. We were standing in his backyard, watching the sun set. His daughter was inside, doing homework. His wife was making dinner.

"Who?"

"Them. My family. When I'm gone. What will they remember about me?"

"What do you want them to remember?" I asked.

"That I was present. That I listened. That I stayed calm when things got hard." He paused. "But I'm not sure that's what they're experiencing right now."

"So change what they'll remember."

"How? I can't just become a different person."

"You already became a different person. In the bedroom. You went from anxious to controlled. From reactive to responsive. From self-focused to partner-focused." I turned to face him. "You know how to transform. You've done it. Now expand the transformation."

He thought about his legacy often now. Every interaction was either a deposit or a withdrawal from his legacy account. Every moment of presence was a deposit. Every distracted response was a withdrawal. Every calm reaction to stress was a deposit. Every irritated outburst was a withdrawal.

His teenage daughter had recently started dating. His instinct was to interrogate, to protect, to control. But he remembered the principles: regulate yourself first. Listen to understand, not to respond. Create safety, not surveillance.

"Tell me about him," he said one evening, keeping his voice curious rather than suspicious. He used the same calm, open presence he had learned to maintain during intimate moments with his wife. No agenda. No judgment. Just genuine curiosity.

His daughter looked surprised. She had clearly been bracing for an interrogation. Then, slowly, she started talking. Really talking. For twenty minutes, she shared things she had never shared before. Her hopes, her fears, her uncertainty about whether this boy really liked her or was just being nice.

David listened. He asked questions that showed he was paying attention. He reflected her feelings back to her. He did not offer solutions or warnings or thinly veiled threats. He simply created a space where she felt safe to be herself.

Afterward, his wife found him in the kitchen, visibly moved. "What did you do? She never opens up like that."

"I listened," David said simply. "I just listened. Like I learned to listen to you."

His wife smiled, understanding. "The TIS thing?"

"The TIS thing," he confirmed. "But it is not really about techniques anymore. It is about who I have become. The kind of man who can hold space for the people he loves."

That was his legacy in the making. Not the construction projects that would eventually crumble. But the feeling of safety he created for the people he loved. The knowledge that they could come to him with anything, and he would be steady. Present. Unshakeable.

His wife moved closer, wrapping her arms around him. "You know what this makes me want to do?" she whispered.

David smiled. The man he had become outside the bedroom was the reason she wanted him inside it. The circuit was complete.

All three men learned the same lesson. And it was John who summarized it best: "It turns out that the man you become outside the bedroom is the reason she wants you inside it."

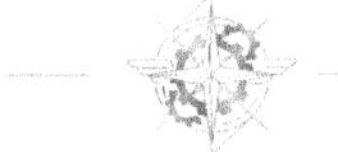

From Masterful Lover to Legendary Partner

Modern relationships do not usually fail because of a single catastrophic event. They erode slowly, worn down by the constant friction of three primary forces: a lack of presence (distraction), a lack of empathy (disconnection), and an inability to manage conflict (reactivity). The skills that underpin the Tactical Intimacy System are a direct antidote to these three forces. You have been training for this without even realizing it. The bedroom was your dojo; the world is now your stage.

Presence vs. Distraction. One of the most common complaints in modern relationships is, "He is here, but he is not here." Think of a couple at a restaurant. He is talking to her, but his phone is on the table, face up. A notification lights up the screen, and for a split second, his eyes flicker down. In that moment, he has communicated a devastating message: *You are not as important as whatever might be on this screen.* The active listening you mastered in Chapter 8 is more than a charisma tactic; it is the ultimate expression of respect. When you give your partner the same undivided focus you learned to apply in the bedroom, you are communicating: *You are my priority. This moment with you is more important than any notification.*

Empathy vs. Disconnection. The effort you put into understanding your partner's pleasure map, learning her rhythms, her cues, her desires, is a training ground for a much deeper skill: emotional empathy. A man who has learned to listen to his partner's body can learn to listen to her heart. Your ability to synchronize with her arousal becomes a metaphor for your ability to synchronize with her emotional states. When she comes home from a brutal day, the *old you* might have tried to solve her problem. The *TIS you* understands that your first mission is not to fix, but to feel with her.

Control vs. Reactivity. We are not talking about controlling your partner. We are talking about controlling yourself. In the heat of an argument, your primal survival instinct will scream at you to interrupt, to defend, to attack, to win the point at all costs. The ability to feel that emotional spike and to consciously take a slow breath for a count of five before you speak, that is a superpower. It breaks the chain of reactivity. You have trained this exact muscle in the most intense and vulnerable environment imaginable. An argument is no match for that level of discipline.

Tactical Drills for Your Partnership

The 10-Minute Undivided Attention Drill. Once a day, commit to giving your partner ten minutes of your absolute, undivided attention. No phones, no

TV, no distractions. Ask her about her day and practice the *Detective* listening style from Chapter 8. Your only goal is to understand her world, not to solve her problems.

The "Translate the Feeling" Drill. The next time your partner is upset or stressed, resist the urge to immediately offer a solution. Instead, try to simply reflect her feeling back to her. "It sounds like you felt completely unseen and unappreciated in that meeting today. That must have been incredibly frustrating." Or: "I hear how worried you are about your mom. It is clear how much you love her." Validating the emotion is often more powerful than trying to fix the problem.

The Conflict Pause Protocol. When you feel an argument escalating, implement the same pause you use during intimate moments. Say: "I need a moment to think about this. I want to respond, not react." Take three slow breath cycles (approximately thirty seconds). Use this time to shift from defensive mode to curious mode. Ask yourself: "What is she really feeling right now? What need is behind her words?" Then respond from that place of understanding.

The Weekly Alignment Check. Once a week, perhaps during your *Money Date* from Chapter 7 or as a separate ritual, ask each other: "What is one thing I did this week that made you feel loved?" and "What is one thing I could do better next week?" This creates a continuous feedback loop that prevents small issues from becoming large resentments.

All three men implemented these drills, each in their own way. John made the 10-Minute Undivided Attention Drill a non-negotiable ritual. Matt mastered the Conflict Pause Protocol. "One breath cycle," he told me. "That's all it takes. One breath cycle before I respond. It changes everything." David embraced the Weekly Alignment Check. "Fifteen years of marriage and we'd never asked each other those questions. Now we have it every Sunday."

Becoming a Legendary Partner and Father

The deepest lesson TIS has taught you is how to manage your own internal state, your impulses, your anxieties, your reactions, in order to create a safe, stable, and predictable space for others. This is the most fundamental duty of a partner and a father.

Your family is your ship, and you are its captain. A captain who panics at the first sign of a storm, who shouts orders based on fear, who gets flustered by chaos, creates a chaotic and terrified crew. But a captain who, in the midst of the storm, the toddler's tantrum, the teenager's rebellion, the unexpected bill, calmly holds the wheel, speaks with a steady voice, and projects an aura of unshakable control, that is the captain his crew will follow anywhere. He makes them feel safe, not because there is no storm, but because he is steady within it.

Your ability to regulate your own nervous system is the greatest gift you can give your family.

Tactical Drills for Fatherhood

The Patience Protocol. When faced with a toddler's tantrum, a teenager's defiance, or a child's endless questions when you are exhausted, implement the same regulation you use during intimate moments. Take one slow breath cycle before responding. This brief pause allows you to choose the Commander's response over the reactive one. Patience is not something you have; it is something you do. It is physiological self-regulation in action.

The Full Presence Play Session. Schedule at least one twenty-minute block per day (or per visit, if you do not live with your children full-time) of completely undistracted play. No phone. No "just checking this one thing." Enter their world completely, on their terms. If they want to play Legos, you are fully engaged in Legos. If they want to tell you about their imaginary world, you are genuinely curious about every detail. This tells them, more powerfully than any words, *You are seen. Your world is important to me.*

The Steady Response Drill. When your child does something that triggers frustration, implement a three-step response: Pause (one breath cycle before speaking). Acknowledge ("I see what happened here."). Respond (address the behavior calmly, without emotional charge). The goal is not to suppress your emotions but to regulate them. Your children are watching how you handle difficult moments. They are learning from your example what it means to be a man in control of himself.

The "I Was Wrong" Practice. When you do react poorly, when you lose your temper or respond with impatience, repair it. Go to your child and say: "I reacted with frustration earlier, and that was not fair to you. I am working on being more patient, and I am sorry. You deserve a dad who stays calm." This teaches your children something invaluable: that strong men can admit mistakes, that relationships can be repaired, and that self-improvement is a lifelong journey.

The Journey Continues: Your Legacy

The Tactical Intimacy System did not just teach you how to control the timing of your orgasm. It taught you the ultimate form of freedom: the ability to act in accordance with your deepest values and intentions, rather than being a slave to your impulses and momentary reactions.

This is what legacy is made of. Not achievements, but character. Not what you accomplished, but who you became.

The ultimate measure of a man is not his momentary victories, but the legacy he builds over time. A legacy is the feeling of safety and respect you inspire in those you lead at work. It is the unwavering confidence and deep sense of being cherished you instill in your partner. It is the quiet strength and patient, undivided presence you offer your children.

The principles you have learned here extend far beyond the bedroom. The Appendix includes resources for continued growth as a partner and father, building on the foundation you have established.

Your legacy will not be measured by how long you "lasted" in the bedroom. It will be measured by how steadfastly you stood as the calm center for your loved ones in the storms of life. It will be measured in the moments of true, undivided presence you gave them. It will be measured by the feeling of safety and unconditional love they felt in your command.

The Tactical Intimacy System has given you the tools to build that steadfastness.

Now, go build that legacy.

For the Seven-Day Presence Challenge, the Legacy Ledger awareness practice, and the complete Connection Toolkit, see Appendix F.

Commander's Q&A: The Life Mission

I have mastered the techniques, but I still feel the pull of my old, impatient habits. How do I make this transformation permanent?

Mastery is not a destination; it is a practice. A black belt in martial arts does not stop training once he gets the belt. Your old neural pathways are like a well-worn path in a forest. Your new TIS pathways are a new trail you are cutting. In the beginning, your brain will naturally want to take the old, easy path. Your job is to consciously and consistently choose the new path, every single day. And on the days you slip up, treat it as data, not failure. Simply course-correct and get back on the new path at the next opportunity. Consistency is the engine of permanent change.

Does becoming this "calm, controlled commander" mean I lose my edge or my passionate side?

This is a critical misunderstanding of control. True control is not about suppression; it is about modulation. A master musician can play a soft, gentle lullaby or a raging, passionate solo. His mastery gives him a wider dynamic range, not a smaller one. By mastering your internal state, you are not killing your passion; you are gaining the ability to unleash it with precision and intent, making it more powerful, not less. You control the fire; you do not extinguish it.

What is the single most important lesson I should take from this entire book?

That you are not at the mercy of your impulses. That your internal state is not something that happens to you; it is something you can actively command. Whether it is the impulse to finish too quickly, the impulse to react in anger to your child, or the impulse to be distracted by your phone, you have learned that there is a space between stimulus and response. In that space lies your power and your freedom. Master that space, and you master your life.

How do I balance being the "calm captain" with being authentic and showing my family my real emotions?

Being a calm captain does not mean being emotionless or hiding your feelings. It means regulating how and when you express them. You can tell your children, "I am feeling frustrated right now, so I am going to take a moment to calm down before we talk about this." This models emotional awareness and healthy regulation. You can tell your partner, "I had a really hard day and I am feeling depleted. I need some time to decompress before I can be fully present with you." This is honest communication. The goal is not to pretend you have no emotions. The goal is to choose how you express them rather than being controlled by them.

When to Seek Professional Help

The techniques in this book are designed for personal development and relationship enhancement. However, there are situations where professional support is essential.

Seek help from a mental health professional if you experience persistent feelings of depression or hopelessness, severe anxiety that interferes with daily functioning, thoughts of self-harm or suicide, or trauma-related symptoms affecting your intimate life.

Consider couples therapy if communication with your partner has broken down significantly, there are unresolved conflicts or resentments, trust has been damaged in the relationship, or your partner is unwilling to engage in the approaches described.

Consult a certified sex therapist if premature ejaculation persists despite consistent practice, there are underlying physical causes that need investigation, or past sexual trauma is affecting your intimate life.

Resources (United States): National Suicide Prevention Lifeline: 988. AASECT (American Association of Sexuality Educators, Counselors and Therapists): www.aasect.org. Psychology Today Therapist Finder: www.psychologytoday.com.

For readers outside the United States: Please search for equivalent mental health, couples therapy, and sex therapy resources in your region. Many countries have national helplines for mental health crises, professional associations for therapists, and directories to find qualified professionals. Your wellbeing matters, and help is available wherever you are.

Commander's Briefing: Chapter 10

- **Your Legacy is Who You Were, Not What You Did.** Achievements are markers of what you accomplished. Your legacy is the feeling of safety, respect, and presence you inspire in others. It is how you made people feel.

- **TIS is a Life Operating System, Not Just a Bedroom Tactic.** The skills you mastered, Presence, Control, and Synchronization, are universal powers. The bedroom was your training ground; the world is now your stage.

- **The Antidote to Relationship Erosion.** Your TIS skills counter the three forces that erode modern relationships: Presence defeats Distraction. Empathy (learned by mapping your partner's responses) defeats Disconnection. Self-Control (mastered in the heat of arousal) defeats Reactivity in arguments.

- **The Captain of a Calm Ship.** The greatest gift you can give your partner and your family is your ability to regulate your own internal state. A calm captain creates a calm ship, even in a storm.

- **Build Your Legacy Through Daily Practice.** The 10-Minute Undivided Attention Drill, the Translate the Feeling practice, the Conflict Pause Protocol, the Full Presence Play Sessions, and the "I

Was Wrong" repair are how you build a legacy one moment at a time.

- **Three Transformations, One Principle.** The bedroom-to-life transfer follows three patterns: extending presence beyond intimate moments into every interaction, applying physiological regulation (breathing, pausing) to family conflict and parenting, and reframing every interaction as a deposit or withdrawal from your legacy account. The skills are identical; only the context changes.

CHAPTER 11

YOUR PERPETUAL MISSION: THE VIEW FROM THE SUMMIT

Six Months Later

THE TEXT ARRIVED ON a Sunday evening, from an unknown number.

"You don't know me, but I know John. He's my neighbor. He told me what you taught him. He said it changed his life. He said it could change mine too. Can we talk?"

I smiled, reading it. John was paying it forward.

Over the following weeks, similar messages arrived. A colleague of Matt's from the hospital. A friend of David's from his construction days. Men who had watched the transformation and wanted the same for themselves.

But the messages that moved me most came from John, Matt, and David themselves. Not asking for help anymore. Reporting progress. Sharing victories. Describing the men they had become.

John's message: "She said yes. I proposed last weekend. She told me she fell in love with me twice, once when we met, and again when I became present. Thank you."

Matt's message: "My son asked me to coach his Little League team. He said I'm the calmest dad he knows. Me. The guy who used to snap over spilled milk. I said yes."

David's message: "Fifteen years of marriage, and she said last night felt like our honeymoon. Not the technique. The connection. Everything we built together. It works."

Three men who started as strangers sharing a common struggle. Three men who are now living proof that transformation is possible.

The View from the Summit

Imagine a mountaineer. For months, he has trained, planned, and struggled. He has battled treacherous ice, punishing winds, and moments of profound self-doubt. And then, he takes the final step. He is standing on the summit. Below him, the world stretches out in breathtaking, silent beauty.

What does he feel? Not an ending, but a new beginning. He sees the world with new eyes. He understands his own limits and his own strength in a way he never could have at the base of the mountain. The climb has fundamentally changed him. The peaks that once seemed impossibly distant are now part of a landscape he understands, a terrain he knows how to navigate.

You have reached the final chapter of this book. You are standing on your summit. But this is not an ending. This is your graduation ceremony, and it is the first official day of your new mission.

You have transformed from a rookie into a pilot, from a pilot into an artist. You have evolved from a reactive machine living in the panicked state of Fight or Flight to a calm commander making conscious, value-driven decisions in Rest and Digest. The Tactical Intimacy System is no longer a tool you use; it is your new operating system.

So, what does a pilot do after he gets his license? Does he hang it on the wall and stop flying? No. He flies. He seeks out new routes, new challenges, and new skies to explore. Mastery is not a destination you arrive at; it is a discipline you live and maintain.

The techniques you have mastered, *The Reset*, *The Breath*, *The Rhythm*, the communication frameworks, the lifestyle tactics, these are not fragile skills that disappear if you stop thinking about them. But they are also not permanent installations that require no maintenance. They are living capabilities that grow stronger with use and weaker with neglect. Your intimate life six months from now, six years from now, will be determined by what you do every day between now and then. This chapter is your operating manual for the rest of your life.

Three Men, Six Months Later

I asked each of them the same question six months after they completed their TIS journey: "What's different now?"

Their answers surprised me. Not because of what they said about the bedroom. But because of everything else. John talked about his relationship. Matt talked about his son. David talked about legacy. The bedroom had been the training ground. The transformation had spread into every room of their lives.

John, Six Months Later

I ran into John at a neighborhood barbecue. He looked different. Not physically, though he was clearly fitter from the morning runs. It was something in how he carried himself. Calmer. More grounded.

"I proposed," he said, grinning.

"And?"

"She said yes. But here's the thing." He paused, choosing his words carefully. "She told me she fell in love with me twice. Once when we first met. And again over the past six months, when I became 'actually present.' Her words."

"How does that feel?"

"Like I almost lost her without knowing it. Like the distracted version of me was slowly pushing her away, and I was too busy looking at my phone to notice. I'm grateful I figured it out in time."

John had made the TIS principles his operating system. The breath cycles that once required conscious effort now happened automatically. The presence that once felt forced had become his natural state. He was not performing anymore. He simply was.

His fiancée had noticed something else: she wanted him more. Not because he had mastered any particular technique, but because the man he had become, calm, present, attentive, was genuinely attractive. The connection they shared now made physical intimacy feel like a natural extension of their daily closeness.

"You know what keeps me up at night?" he said quietly, standing at the barbecue. "Not in a bad way. I lie there after she falls asleep, and I watch her breathe. And I think about how close I came to losing her without ever knowing it. She was right there, every night, and I was staring at a screen. I almost let the best thing in my life slip away because I could not put down a phone." He paused. "I am an engineer. I solve problems for a living. But the biggest problem I ever had was one I could not even see until someone taught me to look up."

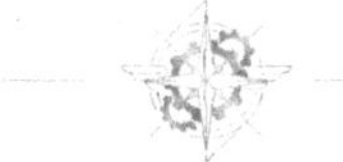

Matt, Six Months Later

Matt called me from the hospital parking lot. I could hear the exhaustion in his voice, but underneath it was something else. Peace.

"My son asked me to coach his Little League team," he said.

"That's great. What did you say?"

"I said yes. But that's not the point. The point is why he asked. He said I'm 'the calmest dad he knows.' Me. The guy who used to snap at him over spilled milk."

"The captain came home."

"The captain came home," he agreed. "And he's staying."

Six months after that devastating question from his son, Matt had transformed his home life. "The Immune" was no longer a title reserved for the operating room. His family, his son and daughter both, now experienced the same steady, calm presence that had saved countless lives at the hospital.

His son had stopped asking whether love meant anger. Instead, he asked something new: "Dad, can we play Legos again tonight?"

Matt said yes. Every time.

His wife had noticed the change in their intimate life as well. "You are not rushing anymore," she observed. "You are not somewhere else in your head. You are here, with me." The techniques Matt had learned were now invisible, integrated into who he was rather than something he did.

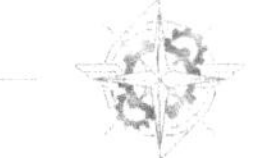

David, Six Months Later

David invited me over for dinner. His wife cooked. His teenage daughter actually joined them at the table, phone put away, engaged in conversation. It was the kind of family scene that feels increasingly rare.

After dinner, while his wife and daughter cleaned up, David and I sat on his back porch.

"You know what I think about now?" he said. "Legacy. What they'll remember when I'm gone."

"And what will they remember?"

He smiled. "A few months ago, I would have said 'the projects I built.' The concrete things. Now?" He gestured toward the kitchen, where his wife and daughter were laughing about something. "That. Those moments. The feeling of being truly seen and heard."

"Your daughter seems different too."

"She still talks to me. That's the miracle. Teenage girl, could easily shut me out. But she comes to me with things. Asks my advice. Tells me about her life." He shook his head in wonder. "I almost lost that. I was so busy being the project manager that I forgot to be her dad."

"And your wife?"

His smile deepened. "Fifteen years of marriage. And she told me last night felt like our honeymoon. Not because of any technique. Because of connection. Because I'm finally the man she married, only better."

"You are different now," his wife observed one evening. "You are the same man I married, but more. More present. More steady. More you."

David smiled. That was exactly the legacy he was building.

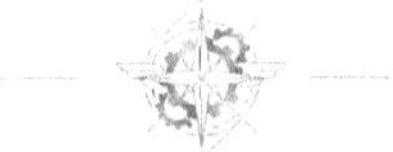

Your Perpetual Mission: The Commander's Standing Orders

This is your standing order. It is the lifelong commitment to live the core principles of TIS every day, in every interaction. The goal now is to transition from *conscious competence*, where you have to actively think about the techniques, to *unconscious mastery*, where these principles become as natural and automatic as breathing itself.

This is not just a poetic idea; it is a neurological reality. The principle of *neuroplasticity* shows that with consistent practice, our brain rewires itself. The neural pathways we use frequently become stronger, faster, and more efficient, literally insulated with a fatty substance called *myelin* that speeds up the signal. They become a well-trodden path in a forest. The pathways we neglect become overgrown and disappear.

Your mission is to walk the TIS path every single day, until it becomes the super-highway of your mind, and the old, muddy paths of anxiety and reactivity are reclaimed by the wilderness.

The ancient Stoic philosophers called this *prosochē*, the practice of constant, vigilant attention to one's own thoughts and actions. Marcus Aurelius, emperor of Rome and one of history's most powerful men, wrote in his private journal every day, reminding himself of the principles he wanted to live by. He understood that wisdom is not something you achieve once; it is something you practice daily. This is the essence of your perpetual mission.

The Three Pillars of a TIS Life

Pillar One: Presence. This is the foundational pillar. It is the commitment to be fully there, not just with your partner, but in your work, with your children, and in moments of solitude. Actively fight the modern disease of distraction. When you are in a conversation, put your phone away, out of sight. When you are working on a task, close the unnecessary tabs. When you are with your children, get down on the floor and enter their world, leaving yours behind. Practice silencing the mental noise and truly listening to the present moment. Make eye contact. Be curious. This is your daily meditation in action.

Pillar Two: Control. This is about conscious self-regulation. It is the ability to command not just your pelvic floor, but your emotional reactions, your time, and your energy. Treat your coherence breathing, a slow inhale for a count of five and a slow exhale for a count of five, as your universal tool, your tactical reset button. Before reacting to a frustrating email, take one cycle. When you feel the spike of anger in traffic, take one cycle. When you feel overwhelmed by your to-do list, take one cycle. This simple act creates a crucial space between stimulus and response, allowing the Commander to make a choice, rather than letting the reactive impulse dictate the outcome. Be the pilot of your values, not a passenger of your impulses.

Pillar Three: Synchronization. This is the pillar of connection. It is the commitment to be a team player not just in the bedroom, but in all areas of life. Actively look for ways to support your partner. If you know she has a stressful day, handle dinner without being asked. Listen to the subtext of her words, the emotion beneath the surface. When you are walking together, consciously match your pace to hers. Learn to breathe in the same rhythm with her, metaphorically and literally, and move together toward shared goals.

The Captain of Your Ship

This book did not give you a fish. It taught you how to fish. More than that, it taught you how to read the map of the ocean, how to understand the weather patterns of your own mind, and how to be the unwavering captain of your own vessel.

There will be storms. Life will throw unexpected challenges at you. There will be days you feel tired, stressed, and tempted to fall back into your old, reactive patterns. That is normal. That is part of the human experience.

Mastery is not about never facing a storm. It is about what you do when the storm hits. It is about remembering the tools you possess, trusting the principles you have internalized, and calmly taking back control of the helm when the waves are crashing over the deck. It is knowing that while you cannot control the wind, you can always adjust your sails.

You are no longer a passenger to your reflexes. You are the captain. You command the ship. You choose the speed, the direction, and the destination. This authority you have claimed over your body extends to every area of your life. The same man who commands his intimate responses commands his emotional reactions, his time, his energy, and his legacy.

John, Matt, and David are now captains of their ships. Not because they never face storms, but because they know how to navigate them. They have the tools. They have the practice. They have the confidence that comes from having already transformed once. And they are paying it forward. Each of them has shared what they learned with at least one other man who was struggling. The ripple effect continues. That is perhaps the greatest legacy of all: not just becoming the man you were meant to be, but helping other men do the same.

This is what you trained for. This is who you have become.

For maintenance protocols, daily drills, and community connection, see Appendix: TIS Digital Resources.

Commander's Q&A: The Lifelong Mission

I have completed the book and I feel great. What is to stop me from slowly losing my motivation and slipping back into my old ways?

This is the most critical question. The answer is ritual and discipline. Motivation is a fleeting emotion; discipline is a system. You must integrate the TIS practices into your daily life until they become non-negotiable rituals, like brushing your teeth. Your morning breathing practice, your weekly check-in with your partner, your daily Undivided Attention Drill, these are the anchors that will hold you fast when the seas of life get rough. And on the days you slip up, treat it as data, not failure. Simply notice what happened, understand why, and course-correct at the next opportunity. Consistency over time matters far more than perfection in any single moment.

Now that I have mastered this, what is the next mountain to climb?

The beauty of the TIS philosophy is that it is scalable to any area of your life. You have learned the meta-skill of conscious, intentional living. You have learned how to master your internal state to produce a desired external result. Now, apply it everywhere. Use the *Commander's Intent* to define your career goals with absolute clarity. Use the *Endurance Tactic* to elevate your health and vitality. Use the *Charisma Tactic* to become a more influential leader and a more connected friend. The Appendix includes resources for continued growth, building on the foundation you have established here. The summit you just climbed was not the only mountain; it was the first, and it gave you the skills and the perspective to climb any other peak you set your sights on.

If you could leave me with one final thought, one single command to carry forward, what would it be?

Be the captain. In every situation, in every interaction, in every moment of choice, ask yourself one question: *Is this action being dictated by my reactive impulses, or is it a conscious choice made by the calm, present commander at the helm?*

The answer to that question will determine the course of your day, your relationships, and your legacy.

You are the captain. Never forget it.

Commander's Briefing: Chapter 11

- **The Summit is Not the End; It is a New Beginning.** Mastery is not a destination you arrive at; it is a discipline you live. This is not a graduation; it is the first day of your perpetual mission.

- **The Mission is Unconscious Mastery.** The goal is to move from *conscious competence* to *unconscious mastery*, where TIS principles are as automatic as breathing. Neuroplasticity is on your side: consistently practiced pathways become your brain's superhighway. The pathways you neglect disappear.

- **The Three Pillars of a TIS Life.** Your perpetual mission is built on three daily practices: Presence (actively fight distraction, be fully there in every interaction), Control (use coherence breathing as your universal reset button for all emotional reactions), and Synchronization (support your partner, listen to subtext, move together toward shared goals).

- **Your Standing Order is "Be the Captain."** In every moment of choice, ask: *Is this action coming from a reactive impulse or a conscious commander?* In the space between stimulus and response lies your freedom and your power.

- **Six Months Changes Everything.** When TIS principles become automatic, three shifts occur: presence extends from intimate moments into every interaction (transforming how your partner experiences you daily), physiological regulation becomes your default response to all stress (not just sexual arousal), and the techniques disappear into who you are rather than what you do. The man you become is the result, not the techniques you perform.

Conclusion: You Are the Captain

Y OU HAVE REACHED THE end of this manual, but you are standing at the beginning of your new mission.

When you first opened this book, you may have been a man living in a state of quiet frustration, a high-achiever paradoxically out of control in one of life's most meaningful arenas. You were the *Apex Predator*, a master of the external world but a victim of your own internal, instinctual programming. Your operating system was running on a program of speed, anxiety, and performance.

Through this journey, you have systematically dismantled that old programming and installed a new one.

You became the *Commander*, learning to set a new intent, one focused on mutual pleasure, not a selfish finish line. You silenced the frantic inner narrator of performance anxiety and replaced it with the calm, curious focus of a detective exploring your partner's pleasure.

You became the *Pilot*, taking firm control of the *Synchronization Engine*. You learned that *The Reset* gives you command over your ejaculatory reflex, that *The Breath* is the remote control for your nervous system, and that *The Rhythm* is the key to managing sensation over time.

You are no longer a passenger to your body's reflexes. You are in the cockpit.

You became the *Artist*, using your control not as a defensive shield, but as an offensive tool to create masterpieces of connection. You learned to amplify pleasure through deliberate control, to explore the vast map of your partner's responses, and to synchronize your experiences into a shared symphony.

And you became the *Legacy Builder*, discovering that these skills, *Presence, Control*, and *Synchronization*, are not confined to the bedroom. They are the pillars of a legendary life. They are the tools you will use to build your legacy as a partner, a husband, a father, and a man.

The *Tactical Intimacy System* is not a set of tricks to be recalled; it is an identity to be embodied. Mastery is not a destination you have arrived at; it is a discipline you will now live. There will be storms. There will be days you feel the pull of old habits. But you now possess the map, the tools, and the training to navigate any terrain.

Viktor Frankl, who endured the worst of human suffering and emerged with the deepest understanding of human freedom, recognized a truth that lies at the heart of everything you have learned: there is a space between stimulus and response.

In that space lies your power. In that power lies your freedom. Whether it is the impulse to release too soon, the impulse to react in anger, or the impulse to be distracted, you now have the ability to command that space.

You are the captain of your ship. Never forget it.

Your mission begins now.

A Final Message from the Author

Commander,

You picked up this book because something was not working. Perhaps it was a source of private frustration, perhaps it was affecting your relationship, perhaps it was simply a gap between the man you knew you could be and the man you were experiencing in your most intimate moments.

Whatever brought you here, I want you to know: the fact that you sought a solution, that you committed to learning, that you did the work, that already sets you apart from most men who simply accept their limitations as permanent.

But I also want you to understand something deeper.

This was never really about lasting longer. It was never about performance metrics or bedroom techniques. Those were just the entry point, the presenting problem that opened the door to something much more significant.

This was always about becoming the man you were meant to be. A man in command of himself. A man fully present with the people he loves. A man whose legacy will be written in the hearts of his partner, his children, and everyone whose life he touches.

The Tactical Intimacy System gave you tools. But you did the work. You rewired the neural pathways. You built the discipline. You became the captain.

I am honored to have been part of your journey. And I am excited for everything that lies ahead for you.

The summit you have reached is not the end. It is the beginning of a life lived with intention, presence, and command.

Now, go live it.

With respect and admiration,

Erdem Ergin Creator of the Tactical Intimacy System

A Personal Request from the Author

If this book has helped you, I would be deeply grateful if you would take sixty seconds to leave an honest review on the platform where you bought this book or use the link at tismethod.com/review

Reviews are the lifeblood of independent authors. They help other men find this system. Men who might be too embarrassed to ask for help. Men who are desperately searching for answers but do not know where to look.

Your review does not need to be long or detailed. Even a single sentence about what resonated with you can make a difference. Your words might be the reason another man finds the courage to take control of his intimate life.

This book exists because I refused to accept that "average" was the ceiling for intimacy. Your review helps spread that message to men who need to hear it.

Thank you for being part of this mission.

With gratitude,

Erdem Ergin Creator of the Tactical Intimacy System

To share your thoughts and help other men discover this system, visit: tismetho d.com

Appendix A: TIS Digital Resources

Your Command Center Beyond the Book

YOU NOW POSSESS THE manual. The techniques, protocols, and frameworks in these pages are complete. Your transformation does not depend on anything beyond this book and your commitment to practice.

What follows is a guide to the digital resources designed to support, accelerate, and deepen that practice.

What You Have Access to Now

As a book owner, the following resources are available to you immediately at tismethod.com/tactical-intimacy/book-owners :

TIS Quick-Reference Field Guide (PDF). A condensed, phone-friendly summary of the essential TIS techniques, drills, and protocols. Designed for fast access during your daily practice or before an intimate encounter. Download it, save it to your phone, and keep it within reach.

The TIS Method Newsletter. Weekly insights on male wellness, relationship health, and personal development delivered to your inbox. Each edition expands on the principles in this book with new research, practical tips, and community perspectives.

Supplementary Resources. A growing library of content that extends beyond the book, including research updates, technique refinements, and guidance on integrating TIS principles into every area of your life.

The TIS Companion App

The TIS Companion App is currently in development. This digital command center is designed to work alongside the techniques you have learned, providing the real-time guidance, adaptive training, and accountability tools that a printed page cannot deliver.

Core capabilities in development include:

Training tools that guide you through the pelvic floor protocol in Appendix E with real-time cues, adaptive progression based on your individual baseline, and streak tracking to maintain consistency. Research consistently identifies adherence as the primary determinant of training outcomes. The app is built to solve this.

A visual Breath Pacer calibrated to the coherence breathing parameters from Chapter 3, synchronized with your training exercises so you are not counting two rhythms simultaneously.

Connection and relationship tools that extend Appendix F into a shared experience with your partner, including scheduling, daily micro-challenges, and communication prompts designed to keep the practices in this book active long after you finish reading.

Lifestyle integration features aligned with the principles in Chapters 5 through 8, supporting the daily habits that build the high-performance chassis for your TIS practice.

Additional modules and features will be announced as development progresses.

Founding Member Access

If you purchased this book before the TIS Companion App launch, you are eligible for **Founding Member** status. Founding Members receive priority access to the app upon launch with a complimentary premium membership period, exclusive to early book owners. This offer is available only to those who register before the app's public release.

How to Register:

Go to tismethod.com/tactical-intimacy/book-owners and enter your name and order number. You will be added to the Founding Member list and receive your Quick-Reference Field Guide immediately.

Your purchase confirmation email serves as your proof of eligibility. For complete terms regarding Founding Member benefits, access duration, and premium membership details, visit tismethod.com/terms.

TIS Method Online

Visit tismethod.com for supplementary resources that go beyond the book, including research updates and a growing library of content on male wellness, relationship health, and personal development. Join the TIS Method community newsletter for weekly insights delivered directly to your inbox.

A Note on Privacy

Your privacy is paramount. The TIS app and website are designed with complete discretion. All personal training data is stored locally on your device and encrypted. Nothing is uploaded to external servers, and no identifying information about your practice is ever shared or visible to others. Your journey is yours alone.

APPENDIX B: TIS PERFORMANCE DRINKS

Targeted Nutrition for Blood Flow and Hormonal Health

THESE FOUR DRINK RECIPES are designed to maximize blood flow, support hormonal health, and deliver concentrated doses of the specific compounds discussed in Chapter 5. They are natural, they are powerful, and they work. You will need a slow juicer (masticating juicer) to make these properly. A centrifugal juicer will not extract juice from leafy greens effectively.

Storage and Shelf Life

Fresh juice oxidizes quickly. For maximum potency:
Best: Drink immediately after juicing.
Acceptable: Store in an airtight glass container, refrigerated, for up to 24 hours.
Not recommended: Storing longer than 24 hours (nutrient degradation).
Fill the container to the very top to minimize air exposure. Add a squeeze of lemon to slow oxidation.

Recommended Progression

If you are new to performance juicing, start with Drink 2 (The Double Shot) for its approachable taste.
Once the habit is established, alternate between Drink 1 (The Vasodilator) for blood flow days and Drink 3 (The Hormone Boost) for hormonal support days.
Add Drink 4 (The Heat) when you are ready for the full experience.
Aim for one drink daily, or at minimum three to four per week, for consistent results.

DRINK 1
"THE VASODILATOR"
Maximum Arterial Expansion

INGREDIENTS

Juice together in a slow (masticating) juicer:

1 medium beetroot (with leaves if fresh)
1 handful of spinach
1 thumb-sized piece of fresh ginger
Juice of half a lemon

WHAT IT DOES

Beetroot delivers massive dietary nitrates, converted to nitric oxide. Spinach doubles the effect. Ginger accelerates circulation. Lemon's Vitamin C extends NO efficiency.

Taste:
Earthy and bold. Ginger and lemon cut the earthiness.

Best For:
Maximum blood flow. The foundation drink.

DRINK 2
"THE DOUBLE SHOT"
Two Pathways to NO Production

INGREDIENTS

Juice together in a slow (masticating) juicer:

1 medium beetroot
1 large slice of watermelon (include white rind)
1 green apple

WHAT IT DOES

Attacks nitric oxide from two angles.
Beetroot provides nitrates (Pathway 1).
Watermelon rind is loaded with L-citrulline which converts to L-arginine then to NO (Pathway 2).

Taste:
Sweet and refreshing. Apple and watermelon mask beetroot.

Best For:
Results without the health-drink taste. Best starting point.

DRINK 3
"THE HORMONE BOOST"
Testosterone and Libido Support

INGREDIENTS

Juice together in a slow (masticating) juicer:

3-4 celery stalks
1 handful of spinach or arugula
1 cucumber
Juice of quarter lemon
Paired with: 1 handful of pumpkin seeds (eaten separately)

WHAT IT DOES

Celery contains androstenone, linked to male hormonal signaling. Spinach provides nitrates. Pumpkin seeds deliver zinc, essential for testosterone production.

Taste:
Clean and green. Cucumber makes it very drinkable.

Best For:
Overall male hormonal health. Ideal daily maintenance.

DRINK 4
"THE HEAT"
Maximum Temperature and Circulation

INGREDIENTS

Juice together in a slow (masticating) juicer:

1 medium beetroot
1 carrot
1 thumb-sized piece of fresh ginger
A pinch of cayenne pepper (start very small)

WHAT IT DOES

The advanced formula. Beetroot opens vessels. Ginger accelerates blood flow. Cayenne's capsaicin causes immediate vasodilation. You will feel warmth within minutes.

Taste:
Sweet, then ginger hits, then cayenne burns. Not subtle.

Best For:
Maximum effect. Graduate to this after Drinks 1 and 2.

Appendix C: Quick Reference Card

Print this page or save it on your phone for fast access during your TIS journey.

The Three Core Tactics

The Reset (Ch3) — Command over the ejaculatory reflex. Before intimacy, perform a series of strong pelvic floor contractions to pre-fatigue the muscle; this primes the reflex pathway and makes in-the-moment Resets more effective. During intimacy, contract your pelvic floor at maximum intensity the moment you feel the warning signs of approaching climax. Hold while breathing. Focus on breath cycles, not seconds: 1.5 cycles (inhale-exhale-inhale) gives approximately 15 seconds, 2 full cycles gives 20 seconds. Feel the reflex retreat. Resume. Three levels: Solo Calibration → Inside Reset (with partner) → Flow State (micro-Resets woven into rhythm).

The Breath (Ch3) — Remote control for your nervous system. Coherence breathing: slow inhale for a count of 5, slow exhale for a count of 5. Continuous cycle. Activates parasympathetic (Rest and Digest) response. Use before, during, and after intimacy. Also your universal tool for emotional regulation in daily life.

The Rhythm (Ch3) — Managing sensation over time. Alternate between shallow and deep movements. Shallow strokes reduce stimulation intensity while maintaining connection. Deep strokes build pleasure. Vary pace and depth based on your arousal level and your partner's responses. The Rhythm creates the wave patterns that synchronize your arousal with your partner's.

Key Frameworks

Commander's Intent (Ch2). Define your mission before every intimate encounter. Your intent is mutual pleasure and connection, not a selfish finish line.

The Synchronization Engine (Ch3). The Reset + The Breath + The Rhythm working as one integrated system.

The Partner's Playbook (Ch4). Your partner is your co-pilot. Communication frameworks: discuss techniques outside the bedroom, establish signals (green/yellow/red), debrief afterward.

The Presence Switch (Ch8). Before transitioning between contexts (work to home, daily life to intimacy), pause. Take five deep breaths. Consciously leave the previous context behind.

Daily Drills & Protocols

Coherence Breathing (Ch3). Daily. 5-10 minutes. Slow inhale for 5, slow exhale for 5. Your foundation practice for nervous system regulation.

Kegel Exercises / Pelvic Floor Training (Ch3). Daily. 5-10 minutes. Progressive contractions building toward maximum intensity holds. The physical foundation for The Reset.

10-Minute Undivided Attention (Ch10). Daily. 10 minutes. No phone, no TV, no distractions. Ask your partner about her day. Your only goal is to understand her world, not to solve her problems.

Full Presence Play Session (Ch10). Daily. 20 minutes. Completely undistracted time with your children, on their terms. Phone away. Enter their world completely.

Conflict Pause Protocol (Ch10). As needed. Approximately 30 seconds. When you feel an argument escalating, say: "I need a moment to think about this. I want to respond, not react." Take three slow breath cycles before responding.

Weekly Alignment Check (Ch10). Weekly. 15 minutes. Ask each other: "What is one thing I did this week that made you feel loved?" and "What is one thing I could do better next week?"

Money Date (Ch7). Weekly or monthly. 30 minutes. Review finances together with equal voice. Align on goals, address concerns, celebrate progress.

Legacy Ledger (Ch10, Appendix F). Daily. 60 seconds. Before sleep, ask: "Was today a net deposit or a net withdrawal?" Based on Gottman's research: maintain a minimum 5:1 ratio of positive to negative interactions. The Legacy Ledger builds the awareness that makes this ratio automatic.

Lifestyle Pillars

Fitness (Ch5). Cardio 3-4 times per week (120-150 minutes total). Strength 2-3 times per week (compound movements: squats, deadlifts, planks). Flexibility: stretch after every workout.

Nutrition (Ch5). Testosterone support (zinc, Vitamin D, healthy fats). Nitric oxide boosters (leafy greens, beets, watermelon). Eliminate saboteurs: visceral fat, smoking, excessive alcohol. See Appendix B for performance drink recipes.

Sleep (Ch5). 7-9 hours per night. Dark room, cool temperature, no screens 30 minutes before bed. Consistent schedule, even on weekends.

Time Management (Ch6). Protect intimate time with the same discipline you protect professional commitments. Quality of presence matters more than quantity of hours.

Financial Health (Ch7). Map your finances. Build an emergency fund. Schedule Money Dates with your partner for financial alignment.

Advanced Tactics (Ch9)

Reset Amplification. Use The Reset at the edge of climax repeatedly to build accumulated arousal. Three levels: Solo Calibration → Partner Integration → Flow State.

Orgasmic Variety. Map your partner's pleasure landscape through curious, non-judgmental communication. Master clitoral, internal, and blended stimulation.

Synchronized Climax. Hold yourself at a high plateau (8-9) using The Reset while communicating with your partner about her arousal level. Time the final ascent together.

Strategic Position Use. Control-focused positions (your safe harbor) for recalibrating. Intensity-focused positions (your advance) when control is confident. Fluid transitions between them.

The Three Pillars of a TIS Life (Ch11)

Presence. Be fully there in every interaction. Phone away. Eye contact. Curiosity.

Control. Use coherence breathing as your universal reset button. One breath cycle before reacting to anything.

Synchronization. Support your partner. Listen to subtext. Move together toward shared goals.

The Standing Order

Be the captain. In every moment of choice, ask: *Is this action coming from a reactive impulse or a conscious commander?*

Appendix D: Recommended Reading

THE FOLLOWING BOOKS INFORMED the philosophy and science behind the Tactical Intimacy System. Each offers deeper exploration of the principles covered in this book.

Mindset and Self-Mastery

Man's Search for Meaning by Viktor E. Frankl. The foundational text on finding meaning through suffering. Frankl's insight that freedom lies in the space between stimulus and response is the philosophical core of TIS.

Meditations by Marcus Aurelius. The private journal of a Roman emperor, practicing daily the art of self-regulation, presence, and intentional living. The original "Commander's Manual."

Thinking, Fast and Slow by Daniel Kahneman. The science of how your brain makes decisions, including the loss aversion and scarcity mindset concepts discussed in Chapter 7.

Relationships and Communication

The Seven Principles for Making Marriage Work by John M. Gottman, Ph.D. The leading research-based guide to relationship health. Gottman's work on conflict patterns and emotional bids underpins the communication frameworks in Chapters 4 and 10.

Hold Me Tight by Dr. Sue Johnson. The science of adult attachment and emotional bonding. Essential reading for understanding the deeper connection dynamics that TIS builds upon.

Come As You Are by Emily Nagoski, Ph.D. A groundbreaking exploration of female sexual response, arousal patterns, and desire. Essential companion reading for understanding your partner's experience.

Physical Performance and Health

Why We Sleep by Matthew Walker, Ph.D. The definitive guide to the science of sleep and its impact on every aspect of health, including hormonal balance and sexual function.

Starting Strength by Mark Rippetoe. The foundational text on barbell training and compound movements. The strength training principles in Chapter 5 build on this approach.

Stoic Philosophy and Daily Practice

The Daily Stoic by Ryan Holiday. 366 daily meditations on wisdom, perseverance, and the art of living. A practical companion for the daily TIS practice described in Chapter 11.

Appendix E: Pelvic Floor Training Fundamentals

Your Eight-Week Protocol for Building the Engine That Powers the TIS Method

IN CHAPTER 3, YOU learned the most important technique in this book: **The Reset**. You experienced its power immediately. A single maximum contraction of your pelvic floor, held before penetration, created a control window you may never have experienced before.

That was your baseline.

This appendix will transform that baseline into mastery.

What follows is an eight-week progressive training protocol designed specifically for the muscles that govern ejaculatory control: the bulbospongiosus and ischiocavernosus.

These are the muscles that contract rhythmically during ejaculation. When they are strong, you can fatigue them at will, disabling the reflex on command. When they are weak, the reflex runs the show.

This protocol requires no equipment, no gym, no special clothing, and no one watching.

Ten minutes a day. Every day. That is all it takes to fundamentally change your relationship with your own body.

> The research supports what you are about to do. A landmark 2014 study at Sapienza University of Rome tracked 40 men with lifelong premature ejaculation through a 12-week pelvic floor rehabilitation program. At baseline, these men averaged less than 40 seconds. After completing the protocol, **82.5 percent** of them gained control of their ejaculatory reflex, and their average time increased to over two minutes. A follow-up study with 273 participants confirmed these results held: **66 percent** of men maintained significant improvement five years later.

This is not wishful thinking. This is progressive muscular adaptation, the same principle that makes your biceps grow when you lift weights. Your pelvic floor muscles respond to training the same way every other muscle in your body does. The only question is whether you will do the work.

Before You Begin: The Ground Rules

Rule 1: Isolate the Target.

The pelvic floor muscles are invisible. You cannot watch them contract in a mirror. This makes it easy to cheat by recruiting larger, neighboring muscles: your glutes, your inner thighs, your abdominals.

If any of these muscles are tightening during your exercises, you are dispersing the effort across the wrong territory. The contraction should be entirely internal, a lifting and squeezing sensation between your tailbone and the base of your penis.

If you have not yet identified these muscles, return to Chapter 3, Section: "Identifying Your Pelvic Floor." The midstream urine interruption test works, but use it only once for identification. Never use it as a regular exercise; repeated interruption of urination can weaken bladder function over time.

Rule 2: Breathe.

Never hold your breath during a contraction. This is the single most common mistake. Holding your breath engages your diaphragm and abdominal wall, which masks the pelvic floor contraction and triggers a sympathetic (stress) response, the exact opposite of what you need. Breathe normally and continuously.

In advanced weeks, you will coordinate your contractions with the coherence breathing pattern from Chapter 3.

Rule 3: Rest Equals Growth.

Every contraction must be followed by a full, deliberate relaxation of equal or greater duration. This is not optional.

Incomplete relaxation between contractions leads to a condition called **hypertonicity**: chronically tensed pelvic floor muscles that are already partially contracted at rest. A hypertonic pelvic floor is closer to the ejaculatory threshold before intimacy even begins.

The relaxation phase is where adaptation occurs. Honor it.

Rule 4: Consistency Defeats Intensity.

Ten minutes of focused daily practice will outperform thirty minutes of sporadic effort every time.

The research is clear: men who train consistently for six to eight weeks report significant improvements. Men who train sporadically do not.

Mark your calendar. Set an alarm. Build this into the non-negotiable architecture of your day, the same way you brush your teeth.

You would not skip brushing for three days and then brush for thirty minutes. The same logic applies here.

Rule 5: Two Types of Contractions, Two Types of Fibers.

Your pelvic floor contains both **slow-twitch muscle fibers** (responsible for sustained holds, endurance, and baseline tone) and **fast-twitch muscle fibers** (responsible for rapid, powerful contractions on demand).

The Reset during intimacy requires both: the sustained pre-fatigue hold uses slow-twitch fibers, and the quick emergency contraction when arousal spikes uses fast-twitch fibers. This protocol trains both, every session, from Week 1.

The Two Exercises

Every session in this program uses two exercises. Master these and you master the protocol.

Exercise 1: The Sustained Hold

Contract your pelvic floor muscles at maximum effort.
Hold for the prescribed duration.
Release fully.
Rest for the prescribed duration.
Repeat.

This trains your slow-twitch fibers. It builds the endurance and fatigue capacity that makes The Reset work.

The goal is to increase both the duration of your holds and the total number of holds per session over eight weeks.

Exercise 2: The Rapid Contraction

Contract your pelvic floor muscles at maximum effort as quickly as you can.
Release immediately.
Repeat in rapid succession at the prescribed tempo.

This trains your fast-twitch fibers. It builds the snap, the ability to fire your pelvic floor instantly when you need an emergency Reset during intimacy.

Think of it as the difference between holding a heavy box (sustained hold) and catching a ball thrown at your face (rapid contraction). You need both.

The Eight-Week Protocol

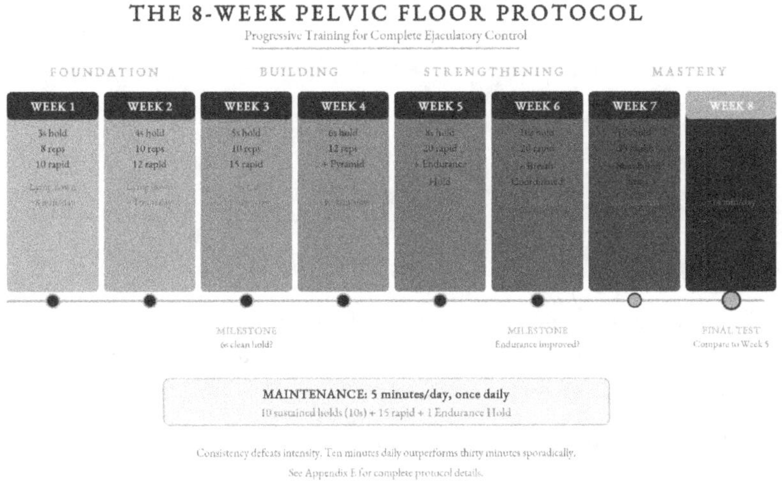

The 8-Week Pelvic Floor Protocol: Overview

Phase 1: Foundation (Weeks 1-2)

Objective: Establish correct technique, build neural pathways, create the habit.

Your primary goal in these two weeks is not strength. It is accuracy. You are teaching your brain to find, activate, and fully release the correct muscles without compensating with your glutes, abs, or thighs. If you rush past this phase, everything built on it will be compromised.

Training Position:
Lying on your back, knees bent, feet flat on the floor.
This position eliminates gravity and makes isolation easiest.

WEEK 1	Phase 1: Foundation Position: Lying down
COMPONENT	DETAILS
Sustained Holds	3-second hold, 6-second rest, 8 repetitions
Rapid Contractions	1-second squeeze-release, 10 repetitions
Sets per Session	3 sets (Sustained Holds first, then Rapid Contractions)
Rest Between Sets	30 seconds
Sessions per Day	2 (morning and evening)
Total Daily Time	Approximately 8 minutes

Execution Notes:

The 3-second hold may feel easy. That is the point.

Focus entirely on isolation. Place one hand on your lower abdomen and one on your inner thigh.

If you feel either tighten, you are recruiting the wrong muscles.

Reset your form and try again.

The 6-second rest between holds is intentional: a 2:1 rest-to-work ratio ensures complete relaxation.

WEEK 2	Phase 1: Foundation Position: Lying down
COMPONENT	DETAILS
Sustained Holds	4-second hold, 6-second rest, 10 repetitions
Rapid Contractions	1-second squeeze-release, 12 repetitions
Sets per Session	3 sets
Rest Between Sets	30 seconds
Sessions per Day	2 (morning and evening)
Total Daily Time	Approximately 9 minutes

Execution Notes:

Increase hold time by one second and add two repetitions to each exercise.

If you cannot maintain a clean, isolated 4-second hold for all 10 reps, stay at Week 1 parameters until you can.

There is no shame in repeating a week.

There is only shame in training the wrong muscles and calling it progress.

Phase 2: Building (Weeks 3-4)

Objective: Increase contraction strength, introduce positional variation, build volume.

You have established the neural pathways. Your brain now knows where these muscles are and how to fire them in isolation. It is time to increase demand.

Training Position:
Sitting upright in a chair, feet flat on the floor.
Gravity now works against you, requiring more effort to achieve the same contraction.
This is deliberate. Intimacy does not happen while lying on your back with your knees bent.

WEEK 3	Phase 2: Building Position: Seated
COMPONENT	DETAILS
Sustained Holds	5-second hold, 5-second rest, 10 repetitions
Rapid Contractions	1-second squeeze-release, 15 repetitions
Sets per Session	3 sets
Rest Between Sets	20 seconds
Sessions per Day	2
Total Daily Time	Approximately 9 minutes

Execution Notes:
The rest-to-work ratio shifts to 1:1.
Your contraction strength should feel noticeably firmer than Week 1.
If you place a finger on your perineum (the area between your scrotum and anus), you should be able to feel a distinct lift during contraction.
This is an excellent way to verify correct engagement.

WEEK 4	Phase 2: Building Position: Seated	NEW: Pyramid Set
COMPONENT	DETAILS	
Sustained Holds	6-second hold, 6-second rest, 12 repetitions	
Rapid Contractions	1-second squeeze-release, 15 repetitions	
Pyramid Set	3s, 5s, 8s, 5s, 3s hold (rest equals hold time after each)	
Sets per Session	2 standard sets + 1 Pyramid set	
Rest Between Sets	20 seconds	
Sessions per Day	2	
Total Daily Time	Approximately 10 minutes	

Execution Notes:

The Pyramid set introduces variable hold times within a single set.

This trains your muscles to sustain effort across different durations, exactly what

The Reset demands during intimacy.

Some Resets are quick 5-second recalibrations.

Others are full 15-second pre-penetration holds.

Your muscles need to handle both.

> **Milestone Check:** By the end of Week 4, you should be able to hold a clean, isolated, maximum-effort contraction for 6 seconds without engaging your glutes, abs, or thighs, and without holding your breath. If you can do this, you are on track. If not, repeat Week 3-4 before advancing.

Phase 3: Strengthening (Weeks 5-6)

Objective: Maximize contraction force, introduce standing position, integrate breathing.

This is where the real transformation begins. You are building the raw strength that will extend your control windows from seconds to minutes.

Training Position:
Alternate between sitting and standing across your two daily sessions.
One session seated, one session standing.
Standing requires your pelvic floor to contract against both gravity and the additional demand of maintaining your upright posture.

WEEK 5	Phase 3: Strengthening Position: Seated + Standing	NEW: Endurance Hold
COMPONENT	**DETAILS**	
Sustained Holds	8-second hold, 8-second rest, 10 repetitions	
Rapid Contractions	1-second squeeze-release, 20 repetitions	
Endurance Hold	1 maximum-duration hold to failure (time it, record it)	
Sets per Session	2 standard sets + 1 Rapid set + 1 Endurance hold	
Rest Between Sets	15 seconds	
Sessions per Day	2 (one seated, one standing)	
Total Daily Time	Approximately 10 minutes	

Execution Notes:
The Endurance Hold is new and critical.
After completing your standard sets, perform one single contraction and hold it for as long as you can maintain maximum effort.
Time it. Write it down.
This number is your benchmark.
It tells you exactly how long your Reset window will last during intimacy.
Track it weekly; it should increase by 2-5 seconds each week.

WEEK 6	Phase 3: Strengthening Position: Seated + Standing NEW: Breath-Coordinated Hold
COMPONENT	**DETAILS**
Sustained Holds	10-second hold, 10-second rest, 10 repetitions
Rapid Contractions	1-second squeeze-release, 20 repetitions
Breath-Coordinated	Inhale (5) contract, exhale (5) maintain, inhale (5) release, exhale (5) rest. 8 reps.
Endurance Hold	1 maximum-duration hold to failure
Sets per Session	2 standard + 1 Rapid + 1 Breath-Coordinated + 1 Endurance
Rest Between Sets	15 seconds
Sessions per Day	2 (one seated, one standing)
Total Daily Time	Approximately 12 minutes

Execution Notes:

The **Breath-Coordinated Hold** introduces the coherence breathing pattern from Chapter 3 directly into your pelvic floor training.

This is the moment where your two core TIS techniques merge.

Your breathing never stops: inhale for five, exhale for five, continuous and steady. Your pelvic floor contracts on the inhale and stays contracted through the exhale, giving you a 10-second hold across one full breath cycle. Then you release on the next inhale and rest through the next exhale.

This is exactly what you will do during intimacy: hold The Reset while breathing continuously to stay calm.

As Matt discovered in Chapter 3, counting breath cycles rather than watching the clock keeps you present with your body rather than anxious about time.

> **Milestone Check:** By the end of Week 6, your Endurance Hold should be significantly longer than your Week 5 baseline. Your 10-second holds should feel sustainable, not maximal. If they still feel like your absolute limit, repeat Week 5-6 before advancing.

Phase 4: Mastery Integration (Weeks 7-8)

Objective: Simulate real-world conditions, integrate all three TIS tactics, achieve training autonomy.

You are no longer just building strength. You are rehearsing the exact muscular patterns you will use during intimacy. This phase bridges the gap between isolated exercise and real-world performance.

Training Position:
All positions. Standing, sitting, lying down, and during movement (walking).
Intimacy is dynamic.
Your pelvic floor control must be too.

WEEK 7	Phase 4: Mastery Position: All positions — NEW: Simulation Set
COMPONENT	**DETAILS**
Sustained Holds	12-second hold, 10-second rest, 10 repetitions
Rapid Contractions	1-second squeeze-release, 25 repetitions
Breath-Coordinated	Full coherence cycle as Week 6. Continuous breathing. 8 repetitions.
Simulation Set	Max hold 15-20s, release 10s, repeat 5 times
Endurance Hold	1 maximum-duration hold to failure
Sessions per Day	2 (vary positions)
Total Daily Time	Approximately 12 minutes

Execution Notes:
The **Simulation Set** is the crown jewel of this protocol.
It replicates the exact pattern of The Reset during intimacy: a sustained maximum contraction followed by a recovery period, repeated multiple times.
Five repetitions simulates a session where you need 5 Resets.
By Week 7, this should feel manageable.
The goal is to reach a point where 3 of these feel effortless, meaning your TIS Level 3 (Proficient) is within reach.

WEEK 8	Phase 4: Mastery Position: All + movement	NEW: Movement Integration
COMPONENT	**DETAILS**	
Sustained Holds	15-second hold, 10-second rest, 8 repetitions	
Rapid Contractions	1-second squeeze-release, 30 repetitions	
Breath-Coordinated	Full coherence integration as Week 7, 10 repetitions	
Simulation Set	Max hold 15-20s, release 10s, repeat 5 times	
Endurance Hold	1 maximum-duration hold to failure (final benchmark)	
Movement Integration	3-minute walk with gentle pelvic floor engagement at 30-40% effort	
Sessions per Day	2	
Total Daily Time	Approximately 14 minutes	

Execution Notes:

The **Movement Integration** exercise trains you to maintain a low-level pelvic floor contraction during physical activity.

This directly prepares you for Level 4 (Master) territory, where micro-Resets become woven into continuous movement during intimacy.

Final Assessment:

At the end of Week 8, record your Endurance Hold time.

Compare it to your Week 5 baseline.

The improvement you see is the physical measure of what you have built. But the real test is The Reset itself.

The next time you use it during intimacy, you will feel the difference.

The contraction will be faster, stronger, and will last longer.

Your control window will have expanded dramatically.

You will be operating from a fundamentally different baseline.

After the Eight Weeks: Your Maintenance Protocol

Completion of this protocol is not the end of your training. It is the transition from building to maintaining. Like any muscle, your pelvic floor will lose its conditioning if you stop training entirely. The good news: maintenance requires far less effort than building.

Your Daily Maintenance Routine (5 minutes):

DAILY MAINTENANCE ROUTINE		
Once daily · Any position · Any time · 5 minutes		
EXERCISE	PARAMETERS	PURPOSE
Sustained Holds Slow-twitch endurance	10-second hold 10-second rest · 10 reps	Preserves fatigue capacity for The Reset
Rapid Contractions Fast-twitch snap	1-second squeeze-release 15 repetitions	Maintains emergency Reset speed
Endurance Hold Weekly benchmark	1 hold to failure Track weekly	Monitors your Reset window over time

Your minimum effective dose. Five minutes preserves everything you built.

This routine continues indefinitely. The path to Level 4 is paved with daily consistency.

Perform once per day, in any position, at any time. This is your minimum effective dose. It preserves the strength you have built and continues the slow, progressive adaptation that will carry you toward Level 4 over the coming months.

Common Mistakes and How to Avoid Them

Mistake 1: Bearing Down Instead of Lifting Up

The correct contraction is a *lifting* sensation, as if you are drawing your pelvic floor upward and inward. The opposite, a pushing or bearing down sensation, is a Valsalva maneuver. It engages the wrong muscles, increases intra-abdominal pressure, and can worsen control. If you feel pressure pushing downward, reset and focus on the "elevator going up" cue: imagine your pelvic floor is an elevator and you are pulling it to the top floor.

Mistake 2: Overtraining

More is not better. Performing four or five sessions a day, or extending hold times beyond what you can sustain with clean form, leads to muscle fatigue without adequate recovery. The result is a weaker, not stronger, pelvic floor. Two sessions per day is the maximum during the eight-week protocol. One session per day for maintenance.

Mistake 3: Ignoring the Relaxation Phase

If you notice a dull ache in your perineum, difficulty fully relaxing after contractions, or a feeling that your pelvic floor is "always on," you may be developing hypertonicity. Incorporate deliberate relaxation practice: after each session, spend one minute in a comfortable position focusing on completely releasing all tension from the pelvic floor. Breathe into your belly. Let everything soften. If symptoms persist, consult a pelvic floor physiotherapist.

Mistake 4: Expecting Linear Progress

Week 5 may feel harder than Week 4. Some days your holds will be weaker than the day before. This is normal muscular adaptation. Strength does not build in a straight line. It builds in waves, with temporary plateaus and occasional dips followed by breakthroughs. Trust the protocol. Trust the science. Do the work.

Your Progress Tracker

Use this simple log to track your development. Record your Endurance Hold time once per week (always at the same time of day, using the same position, for consistency).

WEEK	ENDURANCE HOLD (SECONDS)	NOTES
1		Baseline
2		
3		
4		Milestone Check
5		**First Endurance Hold benchmark**
6		Milestone Check
7		
8		**Final Assessment**

Most men start at 8-15 seconds. By Week 8: 25-40 seconds.
Your number is your number. The only comparison that matters is Week 8 versus Week 1.

The Training Advantage: Why This Protocol Works Better With the TIS Companion App

This appendix gives you everything you need to complete the eight-week protocol with nothing more than a quiet room and a clock. That is by design. Your transformation should never depend on technology.

But there is a reason the world's best athletes do not train alone with a stopwatch.

When the TIS Companion App launches, it will include the **Reset Training Module**: a system designed specifically to accelerate and deepen the work you have started in these pages. The app provides what a printed page cannot:

Real-Time Training Guidance. The app counts your holds and rests for you with visual and audio cues calibrated to each week's exact parameters. You close your eyes, focus entirely on the quality of your contraction, and let the app handle the timing. This eliminates the single largest distraction during pelvic floor training: watching a clock instead of feeling your muscles.

Adaptive Progression. The eight-week protocol in this appendix is designed for the broadest possible range of starting points. The app calibrates to yours. If your Week 1 Endurance Hold is 12 seconds, the app adjusts your target hold times accordingly. If you progress faster than the standard timeline, the app advances you. If you need an extra week at Phase 2, it holds you there without judgment. The protocol adapts to you rather than asking you to adapt to it.

The Accountability Engine. Research consistently identifies adherence as the primary determinant of pelvic floor training outcomes. Men who train daily improve. Men who train sporadically do not. The app tracks your streak, sends discreet reminders at your chosen times, and gives you a clear visual record of every session completed. You will know exactly how many days you have trained, how many you have missed, and what that means for your trajectory.

Coherence Breathing Integration. During Weeks 6-8, the protocol asks you to coordinate your contractions with the coherence breathing pattern. The app's Breath Pacer synchronizes the visual breathing guide with your contraction cues, so you are not attempting to count two separate rhythms simultaneously. One screen. One rhythm. Both systems trained together.

You own this book. The protocol in your hands is complete, evidence-based, and will deliver results if you follow it faithfully. The app, when it arrives, will simply help you follow it more faithfully, more precisely, and with less cognitive effort, the same way a metronome helps a musician practice more effectively than counting beats in his head.

Register for founding member access at tismethod.com/tactical-intimacy/book -owners and receive your free **Quick-Reference Field Guide** immediately while you wait for launch.

> *This protocol is informed by pelvic floor rehabilitation research, including the work of Pastore et al. (Sapienza University of Rome), systematic reviews published in Sexual Medicine and the International Journal of Impotence Research, and clinical guidelines from the Mayo Clinic and Cleveland Clinic. It is designed for educational purposes. If you experience pain during pelvic floor exercises, discontinue and consult a qualified pelvic floor physiotherapist or urologist.*

APPENDIX F: THE CONNECTION TOOLKIT

Practical Exercises, Daily Challenges, and Planning Templates for Building an Extraordinary Partnership

T HE TECHNIQUES IN THIS book taught you to master your body. This toolkit teaches you to master your presence. Every exercise here is designed to create what Dr. John Gottman's four decades of relationship research calls "deposits" in your Emotional Bank Account: the cumulative balance of positive interactions that determines whether your relationship thrives or erodes.

The Research

Gottman's studies revealed that couples who maintain at least five positive interactions for every one negative interaction stay together.

Couples who fall below this ratio do not.

During everyday life, the ratio in thriving relationships is even higher: twenty to one.

A 2020 study in Scientific Reports found that just two weeks of daily mindfulness exercises produced measurable improvements in relationship wellbeing for both the practitioner and their partner.

The exercises in this toolkit are deposits. Each one is small. Each one takes minutes, not hours. And each one, practiced consistently, builds the kind of connection that most couples lose after the first year and never recover.

Part 1: The Seven-Day Presence Challenge

Referenced in Chapter 10. Designed to rebuild your capacity for undivided atten-

tion.

Each day focuses on a single, specific practice. Complete all seven, then repeat the cycle. Within two rotations, these will begin to feel automatic.

Day 1: The Phone Vault

When you walk through the door after work, place your phone in a drawer, a bag, or another room. It stays there for the first 30 minutes you are home. Your only mission: be physically and mentally present with whoever is in front of you. Notice how the first five minutes feel uncomfortable. Notice how the next twenty-five feel different from any evening you can remember.

Day 2: The First-Look Reset

The first time you see your partner today, stop what you are doing. Make eye contact. Hold it for three full seconds. Smile. Say one specific thing you appreciate about them. Not "you look nice." Something precise: "That color makes your eyes look incredible." Specificity is the language of attention.

Day 3: The Detective Listen

At some point today, your partner will tell you something about their day. Your mission: listen without planning your response. When they finish, do not offer advice. Instead, ask one follow-up question that proves you heard the specific thing they said. "You said the meeting felt tense. What made it tense?" Gottman's research: couples who turn toward bids for connection 86 percent of the time stay married. Those at 33 percent divorce.

Day 4: The Unprompted Touch

Three times today, initiate non-sexual physical contact: a hand on the small of her back as you pass in the kitchen, a squeeze of her hand while watching something together, a kiss on the forehead for no reason. Non-sexual touch releases oxytocin, the neurochemical foundation of bonding and trust. Each touch is a deposit in the Emotional Bank Account.

Day 5: The Gratitude Sniper

Send your partner one text message during the day that expresses specific gratitude. Not "thanks for everything you do." Something precise: "I saw that you reorganized the bathroom shelf. I know nobody asked you to do that. Thank you." Research from Florida State University found that expressed gratitude predicted sustained relationship satisfaction over three years.

Day 6: The Full Surrender

For twenty minutes today, do whatever your partner wants to do. Watch their show. Go to their store. Sit with them while they do their thing. No commentary. No subtle signals that you would rather be elsewhere. Full surrender. The message: "Your world matters to me enough that I will enter it completely."

Day 7: The Future Question

Before bed tonight, ask your partner one question about the future: "If money and time were no object, where would you want us to be in five years?" Then listen. Do not solve. Do not plan. Just absorb. You are mapping the terrain of her dreams, the same way you mapped the terrain of her body in the Sensory Mapping Drill.

Part 2: The Charisma Micro-Challenges

Referenced in Chapter 8. Seven daily practices that build the magnetic presence discussed in the Charisma Tactic.

Challenge 1: The Three-Second Pause

Before responding to anything your partner says today, pause for a full three seconds. Breathe. Then respond. This tiny gap eliminates reactive responses and signals that her words matter enough to warrant consideration.

Challenge 2: The Vocal Drop

In your next conversation with your partner, consciously lower your speaking pace by 20 percent. Speak as though every word is chosen deliberately. Research on vocal presence shows that slower speech is perceived as more confident and more attractive. You practiced controlling your rhythm in the bedroom. Apply the same principle to your voice.

Challenge 3: The Specific Compliment

Give your partner one compliment today that she has never heard before. It must be specific and observational: "The way you laugh when you are genuinely surprised, where your whole face changes, is one of my favorite things about you." Specificity communicates attention. Attention communicates value.

Challenge 4: The Story Gift

Instead of reporting your day, tell your partner one moment as a story with a beginning, middle, and end. Include how you felt. Stories create emotional connection. Reports create information exchange.

Challenge 5: The Mirror Move

During a conversation today, subtly mirror her body language. If she leans forward, lean forward. Mirroring signals rapport and empathy. When done consciously, it creates the connection it usually only reflects.

Challenge 6: The Name Drop

Use your partner's first name at least three times today in conversation. Naturally. Research in interpersonal communication shows that hearing your own name activates attention and creates personal recognition. Most long-term couples stop using each other's names entirely. Reverse this.

Challenge 7: The Future Pace

Send your partner a message that creates anticipation for something in the near future. Not a plan. A feeling. "I have been thinking about Saturday night. I have an idea. You are going to like it." Anticipation is a deposit that pays interest.

Part 3: Conversation Starters for Connection Nights

Referenced in Chapter 6 and Chapter 8. Use one per Connection Night. The depth of one question, explored fully, creates more connection than ten questions answered quickly.

1. "What is something you used to dream about that you have not thought about in a long time?"

2. "If you could relive one day from our relationship exactly as it happened, which day would you choose?"

3. "What is something I do that makes you feel safe? And is there something I do that makes you feel the opposite?"

4. "What is the bravest thing you have ever done that nobody knows about?"

5. "If our relationship had a highlight reel, what three moments would be on it?"

6. "What is something you need more of from me that you have been hesitant to ask for?"

7. "When do you feel most like yourself? What are you doing, and where are you?"

8. "What is one thing about your childhood that still shapes how you see the world?"

9. "If you could change one pattern in how we communicate, what would it be?"

10. "What does growing old together look like to you? What does it feel like?"

Rules of Engagement: When your partner answers, your only job is to understand, not to respond, fix, or relate. Ask follow-up questions. Repeat back what you heard.

Part 4: The Legacy Ledger

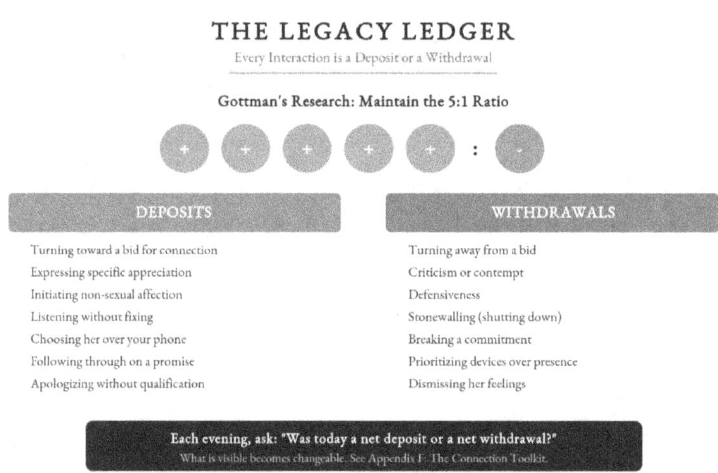

The Legacy Ledger: Deposits and Withdrawals

Referenced in Chapter 10. Based on Dr. John Gottman's Emotional Bank Account research.

The Legacy Ledger is not a scorecard. It is an awareness practice. At the end of each day, take sixty seconds to mentally review your interactions and honestly assess: did I make more deposits than withdrawals today?

What Counts as a Deposit: Turning toward a bid for connection. Expressing specific appreciation. Initiating non-sexual affection. Listening without fixing. Choosing her over your phone. Remembering something she mentioned. Following through on a promise. Apologizing without qualification when you are wrong.

What Counts as a Withdrawal: Turning away from a bid. Criticism or contempt. Defensiveness when she raises a concern. Stonewalling. Breaking a commitment. Prioritizing your device over her presence. Dismissing her feelings.

The Practice: Each evening, before sleep, ask yourself one question: "Was today a net deposit or a net withdrawal?" You do not need to count. You need honesty. If the answer is "withdrawal," you know what tomorrow's mission is.

The 5:1 Target: Gottman's research prescribes a minimum ratio of five deposits for every one withdrawal during conflict, and twenty to one during everyday life. If you are conscious of this ratio, you will naturally begin to course-correct.

Part 5: The Money Date Template

Referenced in Chapter 7. A structured format for the monthly financial conversation.

Before the Date: Both partners review the past month's spending. No judgment. Just data. If either of you is stressed, angry, or exhausted, reschedule.

The Agenda (30 minutes)

Opening (5 min): Each partner shares one financial win from the past month. Start positive. This is a deposit, not an audit.

Review (10 min): Walk through the month's spending together. Use the 50/30/20 framework from Chapter 7. Where did the money go? How does that compare to where you want it to go? No blame for past spending.

Alignment (10 min): Discuss one shared financial goal for the coming month. Specific, measurable, agreed upon by both. Shared goals create shared identity.

Closing (5 min): Each partner shares one thing they appreciate about how the other handles money. End on a deposit. Always.

Rules: No decisions in the moment. Both partners have equal voice. The tone is "us versus the problem" (Chapter 4).

Part 6: The Connection Night Planning Guide

Referenced in Chapter 6.

Step 1: Choose Your Evenings. Block one or two evenings per week. Put them in your calendar with a code name.

Step 2: Create the Transition. Use the Presence Switch (Chapter 8). Close the work chapter. Five deep breaths. Leave devices in another room.

Step 3: Start Slow. Begin with a Conversation Starter, the Breath Synchronization Drill (Chapter 4), or 10 minutes of unstructured time without screens.

Step 4: Remove the Outcome. A Connection Night does not require sex. Remove the pressure of a predetermined outcome, and paradoxically, you create the conditions where intimacy is most likely to emerge naturally.

Your Connection Toolkit at a Glance

Frequency Time Chapter
Seven-Day Presence Challenge *Frequency*: Daily, rotating *Time:* 5-30 min (Ch10)
Charisma Micro-Challenges *Frequency*: Daily, rotating Time: 2-5 min (Ch8)
Conversation Starters *Frequency*: Weekly, *Time:* 15-30 min (Ch6, Ch8)
The Legacy Ledger *Frequency:* Daily (evening), *Time:* 60 seconds (Ch10)
Money Date *Frequency*: Monthly *Time:* 30 min (Ch7)
Connection Night *Frequency:* Weekly *Time:* 1-2 hours (Ch6)

The Digital Advantage: Your Connection Toolkit in the TIS Companion App

Every exercise in this appendix works on paper. But connection involves two people with schedules that conflict and weeks that slip away.

When the TIS Companion App launches, it will include the **Connection Module**:

Shared Connection Calendar. Both partners download the app. Connection Nights, Money Dates, and Presence Challenge days appear on a shared, private calendar. Discreet reminders arrive for both of you. No more forgotten Thursdays.

The Daily Micro-Challenge Engine. Each morning, one Presence Challenge or Charisma Micro-Challenge arrives on your notification screen. The app keeps the rotation running and introduces new challenges beyond this appendix, so the deposits never become predictable.

Legacy Ledger Integration. The evening reflection takes fifteen seconds in the app. A single tap: net deposit or net withdrawal. Over weeks, you see your pattern. The days when work stress creates withdrawals. The weeks when your ratio is strong. What is visible becomes changeable.

Conversation Starter Deck. The ten starters here are your foundation. The app contains over one hundred, organized by depth and category. Your partner can flag questions she wants you to ask her.

Register at tismethod.com/tactical-intimacy/book-owners for founding member access.

> *This appendix draws on the work of Dr. John Gottman and The Gottman Institute, research on mindfulness and relationship wellbeing (Scientific Reports, 2020), and gratitude research from Florida State University. These exercises are for educational purposes. If you and your partner are experiencing persistent relationship distress, consider consulting a licensed couples therapist.*

Glossary: Key Terms Explained

T HIS GLOSSARY PROVIDES QUICK reference definitions for the key concepts, techniques, and terminology used throughout the Tactical Intimacy System.

A

Abundance Mindset. A psychological framework that views resources, including money, time, and opportunity, as plentiful rather than scarce. The opposite of scarcity mindset. Reduces anxiety and enables presence. (Ch7)

Active Listening. A communication technique where the listener focuses entirely on understanding the speaker rather than formulating a response. Involves silencing internal monologue, maintaining eye contact, and reflecting feelings back. The *Detective* approach versus the *Lawyer* approach. (Ch8)

Apex Predator Paradox. The contradiction where evolutionary programming that made men successful hunters (speed, urgency, rapid completion) becomes a liability in intimate contexts where the opposite qualities (patience, presence, extended duration) are required. (Ch1)

B

The Breath (TIS Core Tactic). The second of the three core TIS tactics. Coherence breathing using a slow count of five for inhale and a slow count of five for exhale. Activates the parasympathetic nervous system and maintains calm during arousal. (Ch3)

Bulbocavernosus Reflex. The automatic muscular contraction that initiates ejaculation. The target of The Reset technique, which uses deliberate contraction to fatigue this reflex and prevent involuntary release. (Ch3)

C

Chronos Tactic. The time management strategy from Chapter 6. Named after the Greek personification of time. Focuses on protecting intimate time through morning routines, evening wind-down protocols, and energy management. (Ch6)

Coherence Breathing. The specific breathing pattern used in the TIS system: inhale for a slow count of five, exhale for a slow count of five. Creates approximately six breath cycles per minute, which research suggests optimizes heart rate variability and parasympathetic activation. (Ch3)

Commander's Intent. The psychological reframe from Chapter 2. Shifting the definition of success from "lasting long enough" to "creating a mutually satisfying experience." Changes the mental framework from defensive to intentional. (Ch2)

Cortisol. The primary stress hormone. Elevated cortisol suppresses testosterone and activates the sympathetic nervous system, making control more difficult. Reduced through breath control, sleep, and stress management. (Ch5), (Ch6)

D

Debt Avalanche Method. A debt repayment strategy that prioritizes paying off highest-interest debt first. Mathematically optimal but requires discipline. (Ch7)

Debt Snowball Method. A debt repayment strategy that prioritizes paying off smallest debts first for psychological momentum. (Ch7)

Detective Listening. The active listening approach where the sole mission is to understand. Contrasted with *Lawyer Listening* where the goal is to win the argument. (Ch8)

Dopamine. A neurotransmitter associated with pleasure, motivation, and reward. Builds during arousal and is released in large quantities during orgasm. The Reset Amplification technique allows dopamine to accumulate to higher levels before release. (Ch9)

E

Emergency Fund. Three to six months of essential expenses saved in a high-yield savings account. Provides psychological security that enables presence. (Ch7)

Endurance Tactic. The physical fitness strategy from Chapter 5. Focuses on cardiovascular conditioning, functional strength, and recovery as foundations for intimate stamina. (Ch5)

F

50/30/20 Rule. A budgeting framework: 50% of income for needs, 30% for wants, 20% for savings and debt repayment. (Ch7)

Fight or Flight Response. The sympathetic nervous system activation triggered by perceived threat. Characterized by elevated heart rate, shallow breathing, and muscle tension. The state that leads to loss of control during intimacy. (Ch1), (Ch3)

Founding Member Access. Early book owner benefit providing premium access to the TIS Companion App upon launch. Registration at tismethod.com/tacti cal-intimacy/book-owners. (Appendix A)

Future Pacing. A communication technique that creates anticipation by describing future experiences. Used in building connection throughout the day. (Ch8)

G

Gottman Method. Research-based couples therapy approach developed by Drs. John and Julie Gottman. Referenced for communication techniques including soft start-up and the concept of bids for connection. (Ch4), (Ch10)

H

HIIT (High-Intensity Interval Training). A cardiovascular training method alternating intense effort with recovery periods. Builds the stamina that translates to intimate endurance. (Ch5)

Hypertonicity. A condition in which the pelvic floor muscles remain chronically tensed, even at rest. Results from inadequate relaxation between training contractions. A hypertonic pelvic floor starts closer to the ejaculatory threshold, reducing control. Prevented by honoring the relaxation phase in every training session. (Appendix E)

I

Inside Reset. An advanced application of The Reset technique where the contraction is executed while remaining inside the partner, rather than withdrawing. Requires stronger pelvic floor muscles and greater control. (Ch3), (Ch9)

K

Kegel Exercises. Pelvic floor strengthening exercises named after Dr. Arnold Kegel. The foundation for building the muscular control required for The Reset technique. (Ch3), (Ch5)

L

Legacy Ledger. A daily awareness practice based on Gottman's Emotional Bank Account research. Each evening, assess whether the day's interactions were a net deposit or a net withdrawal. Builds the conscious awareness that transforms the 5:1 ratio from a concept into a lived practice. (Ch10, Appendix F)

Legacy Tactic. The life integration strategy from Chapter 10. Applying TIS principles to become a better partner, husband, and father. Building a legacy written in the hearts of loved ones. (Ch10)

Loss Aversion. A cognitive bias identified by Daniel Kahneman where the psychological pain of losing is approximately twice as powerful as the pleasure of gaining an equivalent amount. Contributes to scarcity mindset and financial anxiety. (Ch7)

M

Micro-Reset. Brief pelvic floor contractions (three to five seconds) integrated into movement during intimacy. Used in Level 3 Flow State to maintain control without stopping. (Ch9)

Mirroring. Subtly matching another person's body language, tone, or pace to build subconscious rapport. (Ch8)

Money Date. A scheduled monthly financial conversation between partners using a structured 30-minute agenda: opening wins, spending review, goal alignment, and closing appreciation. Framed as "us versus the problem" using soft start-up techniques from Chapter 4. (Ch7, Appendix F)

Myelin. A fatty substance that insulates neural pathways, making frequently used pathways faster and more efficient. The neurological basis for why consistent practice leads to automatic mastery. (Ch11)

N

Neuroplasticity. The brain's ability to reorganize itself by forming new neural connections throughout life. The scientific basis for why the TIS techniques become automatic with practice. (Ch11)

Nitric Oxide (NO). A gas molecule that signals blood vessels to relax and widen, directly improving blood flow and erection quality. Boosted through cardiovascular exercise and specific foods including beetroot, leafy greens, and watermelon. (Ch5), (Appendix B)

O

Oxytocin. Often called the *bonding hormone*. Released through physical touch, especially skin-to-skin contact. Builds trust, connection, and attachment between partners. (Ch4), (Ch8)

P

Parasympathetic Nervous System. The Rest and Digest branch of the autonomic nervous system. Characterized by calm, relaxed states. The target state for intimate control, activated through coherence breathing. (Ch3)

Point of No Return. The moment during arousal after which ejaculation becomes inevitable regardless of intervention. The Reset must be initiated before this point to be effective. (Ch3), (Ch9)

Presence Switch. A transition ritual for shifting from work mode to home mode. Involves conscious breathing, intention-setting, and mental closure of work concerns. (Ch8)

Prolactin. A hormone released after orgasm that induces the refractory period and feelings of satisfaction. The Reset Amplification technique delays prolactin release, allowing pleasure to build. (Ch9)

Prosoche. An ancient Stoic practice of constant, vigilant attention to one's own thoughts and actions. The philosophical basis for the perpetual mission of daily TIS practice. (Ch11)

Pyramid Set. A pelvic floor training set with variable hold times (3s, 5s, 8s, 5s, 3s) within a single set, training the muscles to sustain effort across different durations. Introduced in Week 4 of the eight-week protocol. (Appendix E)

R

Reset Amplification. The advanced technique from Chapter 9 that uses multiple Reset cycles at the edge of climax to amplify pleasure and intensify the eventual orgasm. Provides the benefits of traditional *edging* with greater precision and reliability. (Ch9)

Rest and Digest. Common name for parasympathetic nervous system activation. The calm, controlled state required for intimate mastery. (Ch3)

The Reset (TIS Core Tactic). The first and most critical of the three core TIS tactics. A maximum-intensity pelvic floor contraction held for approximately fifteen to twenty seconds (or one and a half to two breath cycles) to fatigue the ejaculatory reflex and restore control. (Ch3)

The Rhythm (TIS Core Tactic). The third of the three core TIS tactics. Deliberate variation between shallow and deep movements to manage stimulation levels and extend duration. (Ch3)

S

Scarcity Mindset. A psychological framework that views resources as limited and threatened. Creates anxiety, defensiveness, and reactive behavior. The opposite of abundance mindset. (Ch7)

Seven-Day Presence Challenge. A rotating cycle of seven daily practices designed to rebuild the capacity for undivided attention: the Phone Vault, the First-Look Reset, the Detective Listen, the Unprompted Touch, the Gratitude Sniper, the Full Surrender, and the Future Question. (Ch10, Appendix F)

Simulation Set. A pelvic floor training exercise replicating the pattern of multiple Resets during intimacy: maximum hold for 15-20 seconds, release for 10 seconds, repeated five times. Introduced in Week 7 of the eight-week protocol. (Appendix E)

Soft Start-Up. A Gottman Method communication technique for raising concerns without triggering defensiveness. Uses "I" statements and focuses on feelings rather than accusations. (Ch4)

Sympathetic Nervous System. The Fight or Flight branch of the autonomic nervous system. Activated by stress, anxiety, or perceived threat. The state that leads to loss of control during intimacy. (Ch1), (Ch3)

Synchronization Engine. The integrated system of The Reset, The Breath, and The Rhythm working together. The core of the Tactical Intimacy System. (Ch3)

Synchronized Climax. The advanced technique of deliberately timing mutual orgasm. Achieved through Reset mastery, communication, and awareness of partner's arousal level. (Ch9)

T

Tactical Intimacy System (TIS). The complete methodology presented in this book. A systematic approach to intimate mastery combining physical techniques, psychological reframes, lifestyle optimization, and relationship skills.

Three Pillars (of a TIS Life). The core principles for applying TIS beyond the bedroom: Presence (fighting distraction), Control (self-regulation in all contexts), and Synchronization (connection and teamwork in all relationships). (Ch11)

U

Unconscious Mastery. The final stage of skill development where techniques require no conscious thought. The goal of perpetual TIS practice. Achieved through consistent repetition until neural pathways become automatic. (Ch11)

DISCLAIMER

Medical Notice

THIS BOOK IS INTENDED for educational and informational purposes only. It is not a substitute for professional medical advice, diagnosis, or treatment. The information provided should not be used to diagnose or treat any health problem or disease.

The author is not a licensed physician, psychologist, urologist, or certified sex therapist. The methods and techniques presented are based on publicly available research, established physiological principles, and educational frameworks, not clinical practice.

If you have or suspect you have a medical condition, including but not limited to premature ejaculation, erectile dysfunction, or any other sexual health concern, consult with a qualified healthcare provider before implementing any techniques, exercises, or lifestyle changes described in this book.

The techniques involving breathwork, pelvic floor exercises, and physical exertion can impact your cardiovascular and nervous systems. If you have a history of heart conditions, high blood pressure, or any urological concerns, consult a qualified healthcare provider before attempting the protocols in this book.

Results Disclaimer

Individual results may vary. The Tactical Intimacy System is a skill-based framework. Like any athletic or cognitive discipline, results depend on individual physiology, consistency of practice, and adherence to the system.

No guarantees are made regarding the effectiveness of any technique or strategy presented in this book. Factors including underlying medical conditions, medications, psychological state, and relationship dynamics can significantly affect outcomes.

Relationship Notice

The partner communication strategies in this book are general guidelines for healthy relationships. If you are experiencing significant relationship difficulties, communication breakdowns, trust issues, or if your partner is resistant to the approaches described, consider seeking guidance from a licensed couples therapist or relationship counselor.

Mental Health Notice

If you are experiencing symptoms of depression, severe anxiety, thoughts of self-harm, or any mental health crisis, seek help from a qualified mental health professional immediately.

The stress management and mindset techniques in this book are designed for general personal development. They are not intended to diagnose or treat clinical mental health conditions.

Crisis Resources

988 Suicide and Crisis Lifeline: Call or text 988 (US)

Crisis Text Line: Text HOME to 741741 (US)

For readers outside the United States, search for equivalent crisis resources in your region.

Fitness and Nutrition Notice

Before beginning any exercise program or making significant dietary changes as suggested in this book, consult with your physician, especially if you have pre-existing health conditions, are taking medications, or have concerns about your physical health.

Case Studies Notice

The case studies in this book are based on real individuals whose names and identifying details have been changed to protect their privacy. Any resemblance to other specific individuals is coincidental.

Legal Acknowledgment

By reading and using this book, you acknowledge that you have read, understood, and agree to this disclaimer. The author and publisher disclaim any liability for any adverse effects arising from the use or application of the information contained herein.

ACKNOWLEDGEMENTS

THIS BOOK EXISTS BECAUSE three men trusted me with their most private struggles. John, Matt, and David (not their real names) allowed me to share their journeys so that other men could benefit from what they learned. Their courage, honesty, and willingness to grow made this book possible. I am grateful beyond words.

To my family, whose patience and support gave me the space to write. You are the reason I understand what legacy truly means.

To the researchers, clinicians, and thinkers whose work informed this book, from John Gottman's insights on relationships to Viktor Frankl's wisdom on human freedom to Marcus Aurelius's enduring lessons on self-mastery to the countless scientists advancing our understanding of male sexual health. I stand on the shoulders of those who came before.

To every man who picks up this book and decides that he is worth the effort of transformation. You are already ahead of most. The fact that you are here, reading these words, means you have the courage to change. That courage is the foundation upon which everything else is built.

And to the partners of the men who read this book. Your patience, your honesty, and your willingness to be part of the journey make all the difference. This book is for both of you.

About the Author

Erdem Ergin is the creator of the Apex Predator Paradox and the architect of the Tactical Intimacy System (TIS Method), the first performance framework that treats male intimate control as an engineering problem, not a psychological weakness.

His work combines neurobiology, tactical discipline, and relationship science.

Years of research revealed a hidden pattern: the most driven and successful men are statistically most susceptible to losing control in their intimate lives.

The same neural wiring that makes a man unstoppable in business is the exact programming that sabotages him in the bedroom. He named this the Apex Predator Paradox, and it affects one in three men.

Applying systems-based thinking to the one domain nobody had properly systematized, Erdem created the TIS Method: a complete operator's manual built on neuroscience, Gottman's relationship research, and physiological tactics that give men real, mechanical control.

His flagship book, Tactical Intimacy: The TIS Method, goes far beyond the bedroom. Across 11 chapters, it delivers a full operating system covering physiological control, partner communication, fitness protocols, and the stoic philosophy of intentional living.,

It is written for the analytical mind, the man who optimizes his sleep, training, and portfolio but lacks a system for his most crucial relationship.

Erdem also publishes the TIS Intel Briefing, a regular newsletter for men committed to presence, control, and connection, and shares tactical insights globally under the TIS Method brand through www.tismethod.com, where you can join the newsletter, access supplementary materials, and follow the TIS Method on social media. @TISMethod

For speaking inquiries, media requests, or partnership opportunities, contact: info@tismethod.com